'00

4-

Holy HORMONES!

APPROACHING PMS & MENOPAUSE GOD'S WAY

J. Ron Eaker, M.D.

Printed in the United States of America

Packaged by Selah Publishing

ISBN 1-58930-000-9
Library of Congress Catalog Card Number: 99-90629

DEDICATION

To God, who is the Great Healer, and to His Glory.

To the women in my life who taught me love, respect, and faith: Dot Bouldin (Mom), my wife Susan, and our daughters Katie and Caroline. This book would not have been written if it weren't for their encouragement, teaching, compassion, tolerance, and unending love.

To my in-laws, Dr. and Mrs. William C. Shirley, who not only share their most precious possession, their beautiful daughter, but who also continue to inspire me as a physician. Bill is a man truly in love with the wonder of medicine.

And finally, to my patients: May they read, take action, and learn to celebrate life and all God has provided.

ENDORSEMENTS

"Ron Eaker has given us a road map to healthier, happier living. Wise and witty, frank and faithful, Ron weaves medicine and religion together, as God surely intended them to be. Then step by step, he invites the reader to move in the right direction. I recommend his book to any woman who is dealing with PMS or menopause? and to the man who loves her!"

—Dr. David Jones

Senior Pastor, Trinity-on-the-Hill United Methodist Church, Augusta, GA

"When hormonal issues hit us, our usually cheerful countenance becomes a fearful confusion. We feel more hostile than holy; ashamed of our actions, uncomfortable with our bodies, and too embarrassed to ask for help. In one comprehensive guide, Dr. Eaker provides women of all ages hope for their female concerns."

—Marita Littauer

President, CLASServices Inc.

I found this book to be truly informative, spiritual, and humorous...Dr. Eaker uses the Bible to show us that God does have a plan in PMS and Menopause... [Dr. Eaker] is quick to point out that WE control our way of thinking...He shows us some very realistic goals, and how to best achieve them, by taking them one at a time! Dr. Eaker is quick to offer advice on methods for dealing with PMS and menopause ... (including) hormonal therapy ... herbs, diet, ... [and] our spiritual well being. He is a wealth of information on other sources to gather the information we seek: the Bible, other publications, and of course, the Internet ... Thank you, Dr. Eaker, for helping me to see the things that were just beyond my view, and teaching me what I need to do to help myself through PMS ... [toward] the glory that can be found in menopause!

—Darci Warner

ParentClub.com

ACKNOWLEDGMENTS

Every project, every mission, every passion, has champions. This project is no exception. Without these champions, this book would still be just a wish, relegated to the " what if" file of my brain. It is a true joy to express my thanks to these individuals, even before they croak!

My dad, who is still wondering what all the hoopla is about.

Marita and Florence Littauer and CLASS Services for inspiration and encouragement.

My Emmaus brothers and prayer warriors, Don and Andrew.

Deb Strubel for her behind the scenes editing which actually made the manuscript readable.

My Partners, Dr. G. Pat Williams, Dr. Sarah Speese, and Dr. Kerry Kline who allowed me to be gone far too often.

David Jones for his guidance, teaching, and friendship.

Jacqueline Cromartie and the staff at Jakasa for believing and helping me get the word out.

Kathleen Jackson, a woman who loves Jesus and lives her beliefs, for giving me a platform.

Kay-Lynn Chritton and her staff at K.C. Productions for their creative passion, belief in the message, and willingness to go beyond to continually acheive excellence.

CONTENTS

SECTION 4
Bouncing, Binging, Bones, and Believing

DISCLAIMER

This book's goal is to provide you with information that may be useful in attaining optimal health. Nothing in it is meant as a prescription or as medical advice. You should check with a physician or other health care provider before implementing any changes in your lifestyle, especially if you have physical problems or are taking medication of any kind. Many of the products mentioned in this book are described by their tradenames. The companies that make the products claim these designations as legally protected trademarks. It is not our intent to use any of these names generically, and the reader is cautioned to investigate a claimed trademark before using it for any purpose except to refer to the product to which it is attached.

Another PMS and Menopause Book?

Menopause is not a disease. Let me repeat, menopause is not a disease. PMS is not all in your head. I consider myself an optimist (some say I am just a pessimist who doesn't know better), and my approach to PMS and menopause is one of expansive idealism. I debated *ad nauseam* about beginning a book with such a negative pronouncement. Yet in this particular case I wanted to establish an important thesis at the very beginning. The concept of menopause as the "ultimate and inevitable bad experience" is so pervasive in this culture that I must challenge it from the outset. This is the tone for the chapters to come. This is the theme that will be repeated. God did not design women to self-destruct at fifty! If you remember little else from this book please remember this: Menopause is a normal, natural transition, not a disease.

Origins

Midlife and menopause *are* many things. In my role as an obstetrician and gynecologist I have heard them labeled everything from a wake-up call to a dead-end street. Because this book is based on the Word of God, I won't use some of the "colorful" descriptions of menopause that have been volunteered to me over the years. Confusing, challenging, exciting, disappointing, illuminating, frustrating, and promising. This smorgasbord of feelings, thoughts, and beliefs defines the menopausal experience.

As a physician, my approach to midlife and menopause over the past sixteen years of practice has been fairly simple: This is a normal, natural transition that is individually experienced. There are some universal similarities, but because of every woman's unique physiology and life experiences, this time in a person's life is unpredictable. What your mother experienced, or what Aunt Jessie next door felt, impacts little or none on your menopause. It doesn't follow the rulebook; in fact there is no rulebook. But there is a guidebook. I believe the Bible embodies all the wisdom one needs to celebrate menopause. I believe that the Bible lays the foundation for a house of stone to weather the midlife storms. As Jesus said in the Gospel of Luke, "It is like a person who builds a house on a strong foundation laid upon the underlying rock. When the floodwaters rise and break against the house, it stands firm because it is well built. But anyone who listens and doesn't obey is like a person who builds a house without a foundation. When the floods sweep down against that house, it will crumble into a heap of ruins." (Luke 6:48–49)

Contained in the sacred pages of the Old and New Testaments are instructions that are easily applied to midlife changes, PMS, and menopause. Barricade yourself from the tribulations of midlife. Establish your foundation in the wisdom and guidance of the Word.

In the pages that follow I illustrate how the Bible has a plan for this time in your life. There are no "Ten Commandments" of menopause, yet the wisdom and guidance that can be gleaned from both the Old Testament and the New Testament can be applied daily to *your* life. Tom Minnery, writing in *Christianity Today*, said, "[When] I was younger, I tended to believe that certain principles were true because they were in the Bible. But year by year, as I have read much of the social research, I have come to look at this a new way—that certain principles are in the Bible because they are true. They are true and helpful for all people, regardless of whether they accept or reject the Bible's central claim." These enduring biblical principles provide daily safe paths to walk in your search for contentment in the midst of transition.

I am a "recovering traditionalist." I was trained in the old-school approach to menopause—which means drugs and, if that didn't work, more drugs. I quickly discovered that this philosophy was not only very limiting but also possibly dangerous. I learned this truth not in the textbooks or the halls of academia, but through the patients I worked with.

Imagine the surprise and confusion of a young doctor learning . . . from his patients! I once again became a student, learning from others what only they could impart, because they lived it! I began to understand that a person who learns only from himself has a fool for a teacher. These wonderful and courageous women taught me that the common approach to dealing with menopausal symptoms was occasionally successful. However, women were not satisfied with their options, and many discovered that the treatment was worse than the symptoms.

One lady put it well: "Physicians have a duty to give a woman the best care they can provide. However, each person is ultimately responsible for his or her own health. We, the patients, need help, guidance, and a listening ear." That has become my charge, and the charge of this book: To do the best I can with my knowledge base in providing help, guidance, and most importantly, a listening ear. But I didn't forget the other point she made. *Your* health is *your* responsibility. Those are powerful and challenging words.

The Problem

My perception of a general dissatisfaction among women was confirmed as I read that only 17 percent of eligible women in the United States were taking some type of hormone replacement and up to 80 percent of women who started on hormones had stopped them after two years![1] It was not hard to understand that something was wrong. The groundswell was beginning to resonate. The needs of women were not being met. If three-quarters of the people who started insulin treatment for diabetes stopped it, they would be in a mess. Likewise, if you believed the premise that hormones were essential to health and almost three-fourths of the women who began them stopped them, then we were setting ourselves up for a major health crisis. I was not seeing this develop in my own practice.

I began to question the caveat that hormones were essential to postmenopausal health. And if they weren't used, were there complementary therapies available as viable options? To answer those questions I embarked on a self-study program to look at what I could offer. I could not find a single text that combined my deep foundational beliefs in God's Word and my desire to provide options to women with regards to their menopausal experience. As Paul wrote in his letter to the Romans, "Such things were written in the Scriptures long ago to teach us. They give us hope and encouragement as we wait patiently for God's promises." (Romans 15:4) I learned from patients who were on this journey; in fact, many have been my fellow travelers along this road and are still learning with me today. It is an ongoing process.

Biblical Guidance

I understood long ago that the best textbook for living is the Bible. It is the user's manual that we can apply from birth to the grave. Abraham Lincoln said, "This great book [the Bible] is the best gift God has given to man. But for it, we could not know right from wrong." I understood this concept as it applied to my life, but I was slow to translate this into how I cared for patients. If the words and teachings in Scripture are a template upon which to pattern life, then why couldn't these same instructions be applied to the women I saw every day struggling with issues of midlife? The obvious answer was that they most certainly could.

This didn't come quickly to me. I tend to be slow to hear with my spiritual ear, yet God's persistent voice finally broke through my barriers. It was one of those "ah-ha!" moments. I had been doing lectures and seminars for years on alternative approaches to menopause, yet I felt the message was incomplete. While I was working on a talk about the healing power of prayer, an old slide from a previous menopause talk somehow got mixed in the tray and the connection was made. (Some say coincidence is just God's way of remaining anonymous.) God is a healing God, and here I was dealing with countless women who were in need of healing of mind, body, and spirit. What a perfect fit!

I am now convinced that it is the only way all the pieces can fit. These women fighting with change-of-life issues had all the knowledge about traditional medical and alternative approaches, yet they were still struggling to achieve an internal peace. What was missing was the third component, the spirit. What was keeping my patients from experiencing real joy and peace during this transition was the guidance and assurance of Scripture.

Dr. S. I. McMillen wrote in his fascinating book, *None of These Diseases*, "Obedience to Biblical precepts is still one of the most effective ways to prevent many of the afflictions of mankind."[2]

Health and Christian theology are so intertwined that I thought there would be a wealth of resources available with specific biblical insights for dealing with the physical and emotional changes of menopause. I began looking for books that described a biblical approach to midlife. I searched extensively, using all manner of queries. I came up empty-handed. Even on the information superhighway, the Internet, I was unable to locate any comprehensive resources that adequately addressed this topic. There were a multitude of books, tapes, and videos on menopause and volumes on complementary approaches. However, I was unable to find any comprehensive book that specifically looked at biblical principles as applied to midlife and menopause. Thus the idea for this book grew out of a need for a reference to guide patients who wanted a biblically-based, scientifically-correct, practically-applied guide to midlife and menopause.

This book was conceived through much prayer and help from many people. The labor was intense and the birth painful, yet just as in childbirth, the result was rewarding.

Natural Approach

My bias is to look at "natural" ways of approaching the menopause. I believe God has bestowed on us all the tools to live healthy, happy productive lives. Information on herbs, complementary teachings, prayer, diet, and exercise will help. But I also know that, for some, conventional approaches to this transition (especially when it comes to symptom treatment) are useful and successful. My background is in traditional medicine, and I know that this is of God. This book is about choice and responsibility, both of which are sound biblical principles. The New International Version of the Bible has 78 listings for the word *choice*. The twelfth chapter of Romans spells out the importance of personal responsibility. God has provided many paths to a joyous menopause; you must choose your path. This book is about giving you the options, detailing the consequences, and prodding you to action.

The major problem in meshing traditional and complementary approaches to health is a mistaken perception of mutual exclusivity. This is a sad and limiting assumption because it blocks many from understanding the options God has provided. These apparently diverse approaches actually are intertwined when a truly biblical application is sought. I do not presume to say God ordains only "natural" approaches versus "traditional" approaches. The arrogance of that is obvious.

I am saying that choice and personal responsibility are keys to unlock a joyous menopause, and this book helps you choose the right key for your lock. Some misinformed individuals feel that if you approach health with only "traditional" solutions of modem medicine you are "taking the easy way out" or "polluting your body." Likewise, if you shun conventional medicines in favor of herbs and home remedies you are labeled a "wacko earth mother" by the conventional medical establishment. These characterizations reflect more on the accusers than the accused. I have met just as many close-minded "naturalists" as I have open-minded "traditionalists." The secret is balance. I believe both approaches can be of God.

There is a profound misperception that science and the Bible are not compatible. The reality is that the two are complementary. The 1972 General Conference of the United Methodist Church issued a statement in one of its documents that said, "All truth has its source in the God of truth so that our efforts to discern the connections between faith and science, grace and nature, are useful endeavors in developing credible and communicable doctrine." The relationship between science and the Bible has spawned debate and scholarly works for centuries. Hebrews 11:3 states, "By faith we understand that the entire universe was formed at God's command, that what we now see did not come from anything that can be seen."

Science and all that it encompasses is part of the natural universe; therefore, science is of God. The prime assumption is that God is the author of creation. Understand that I am not equating science with "traditionalism" and the Bible with "naturalism" and thereby staging a pseudo competition between right and wrong. This is an attempt to show that "in the beginning was the Word," and that authority extends today in matters of life and health. Without that understanding the entire premise of this book is invalid. *Time* magazine for March 5, 1990, carried an article by Michael D. Lawrence concerning new evidence about the fall of Jericho. Lawrence said, "In matters of faith, science can never provide the ultimate answers." *Faith* and *fact* will provide the woman facing midlife with an unbeatable combination.

Dr. McMillen writes, "Medical science is still discovering how obedience to ancient prescriptions saved the primitive Hebrews from the scourges of epidemic plagues; and medical research is constantly proving the timeless potency of the divine prescription for modern diseases."[3]

My themes for this book are multiple yet simple. First, menopause is a normal change. Second, God has a plan to allow you to truly celebrate any change. Third, there are choices that every woman needs to make and important questions that must be answered. This is an opportunity to live with passion and fulfill your mission, a mission that is not completed until the Lord decides it is time to come home. I read once of a famous preacher who was asked when he thought his purpose in life would be achieved. He replied, "If I am still breathing, it hasn't been!"

This is a time to take stock of the past and choose your path for the future. The choice is yours. It is a choice that is difficult, if not impossible, to make wisely without sound information and guidance. In medicine and surgery we have a ritual called informed consent. It is a process whereby a patient contemplating a surgical procedure is told of all the potential complications and alternatives to that procedure. It is then the patient's responsibility to ask any questions she may harbor, and then, based on all this information, consent to the procedure. This book is like an informed consent for menopause and PMS. You will be presented with a great deal of information, yet the final decision on action is yours.

SECTION ONE

Laying the Foundation

CHAPTER ONE

The Healing Triad

"I'm falling apart, and I don't know how to put all the pieces back together."

Shelly was nearly at the end of her rope, and sliding fast. She was a slightly obese woman in her late forties who was looking for answers, quickly. "My biggest two problems are that I have no energy and absolutely no sex drive," Shelly told me. "Even when I do feel good, I would rather knit than make love. My husband likes sweaters, but not that much!"

I was relieved that Shelly still had her sense of humor. She was going to need it! For Shelly to become whole, she needed to approach her situation from three separate, yet related, directions. She had to look at her problems not as isolated afflictions but as opportunities to explore her mind, body, and spirit.

As it turned out, Shelly was fatigued from her hypertension medication. She also suffered from painful intercourse, which led to her libido problems. Furthermore, during her initial exam, she revealed that an uncle had sexually abused her when she was eleven, and she had never been able to tell any family members about her trauma. She was a deeply religious woman but was having great difficulty relating her Christian beliefs and her physical complaints.

The solutions to Shelly's problems were not in simply changing her blood pressure medication and giving her estrogen to increase vaginal lubrication. These approaches may be appropriate, yet they only address one aspect of Shelly: her physical body.

To become healed (whole), Shelly must balance her body with her mind (beliefs, thoughts, and emotions) and her spirit (her relationship with God). To ignore any component of this healing triad would be to rob Shelly of true wellness.

Shelly's healing path began with an understanding that she was not defined by her maladies. She was a child of God, intrinsically healthy, who was temporarily out of balance.

Health for Shelly, and for each of us, is not just the absence of disease. It is much more than that. The word originally meant "to make whole," and this embodies my perception of the essence of health. A healthy person is one who strives for a balance among all the components of wellness. Those components are the healing triad: mind, body, and spirit.

For the first several years of my medical practice, I focused exclusively on the health of the physical body. Through my interaction with patients I began to appreciate the powerful influence of thoughts, emotions, and feelings on health. We are what we think. This dualism of mind and body was more congruent with my concept of healing. However, I began to experience a sense of incompleteness with this approach.

I was seeing many women who were in excellent physical health and mentally acute, yet they were in pain. It was an emotional pain that burrowed deep into their hearts. It was a pain that arose from their innermost being, their soul. These were people who were struggling with the third component of wellness, that of the spirit. Being physically fit and mentally sharp was not enough. Only by filling this spiritual void could a balance be achieved. To fully realize your health potential, you must seek and feed this universal spiritual hunger. The Bible feeds this hunger with its guidance, wisdom, and practical advice.

There is an intimate connection among these three entities (mind, body, and spirit) that links their purpose. It is like a mobile hanging over a baby's crib. If you pull on one part of the mobile, all of the others move in response. So it is with health. A change in your physical body will impact how you feel emotionally. I believe it is hard to achieve balance and contentment in your physical and emotional health if your spiritual life is not healthy. (This is not a new concept.)

Paul reflects on the importance of this healing triad in his letter to the Thessalonians. "Now may the God of peace make you holy in every way, and may your whole spirit and soul and body be kept blameless until that day when out Lord Jesus Christ comes again" (2 Thessalonians 3:16). Again Paul, in his letter to the Romans, expressed this integration of entities. "And so, dear brothers and sisters, I plead with you to give your *bodies* to God. Let them be a living and holy sacrifice—the kind he will accept. When you think of what he has done for you, is this too much to ask? Don't copy the behavior and customs of this world, but let God transform you into a new person by changing the way you *think*. Then you will know what God wants you to do, and you will know how good and pleasing and perfect his will really is."(Romans 12:1–2, emphasis mine).

And in Matthew 22:37–38 Jesus responds to the question, what is the greatest commandment, by stating, "'You must love the Lord your God with all your *heart*, all your *soul*, and all your *mind*. This is the first and greatest commandment."(emphasis mine)

Comfort

No matter how well you prepare, there will come a time in the race through midlife that you experience pain and frustration, and you will ask yourself, do I have the will to go on? Maybe, less dramatically, you will ask, how can I best go on? The answer lies in your training. What is the foundation that supports you in hard times? What is it that carries you those last few miles when you want so desperately to quit? Better yet, what is it that gives you the ability, confidence, and wisdom to breeze through challenges? Only your applied knowledge, experience, and faith can provide these resources.

You can run the race knowing that it will be fraught with ruts and roadblocks; however, you can be secure in knowing that you are not running alone. This is where learning about physiology and medicines falls short. Midlife and menopause can only be lived joyously when there is a balance of mind, body, and spirit. If you only focus on the mind and the body, you will miss the comfort of the Spirit. There is comfort in the Word. There is comfort in knowledge. Nowhere is this comfort better illustrated than in the twenty-third Psalm.

> The Lord is my shepherd; I have everything I need.
> He lets me rest in green meadows; (*even with hot flashes*)
> He leads me beside peaceful streams. (*in the middle of night sweats*)
> He renews my strength. (*when fatigue takes over*)
> He guides me along right paths, bringing honor to his name. (*showing me options*)
> Even when I walk through the dark valley of death,
> I will not be afraid, for you are close beside me. (*depression cannot rule me*)
> Your rod and your staff protect and comfort me. (*herbs and vitamins, too*)
> You prepare a feast for me in the presence of my enemies.
> You welcome me as a guest, anointing my head with oil. (*flaxseed, chamomile*)
> My cup overflows with blessings. (*At least I am here to experience menopause, the other option is not so great*)
> Surely your goodness and unfailing love will pursue me all the days of my life,
> and I will live in the house of the Lord forever. (*wrinkles and all*)

Menopause Explosion

The shelves at the local bookstore are bursting with "how to" and "how not to" books on menopause. Menopause has come out of the closet. Just a few years back it was impossible to find any books solely devoted to menopause. Just asking the clerk or librarian brought smirks or hushed murmurs. "We don't have much on *that* subject, dear." It was if you had to wear a giant scarlet M on your dress to signify you were a wayward woman for wanting information. Gail Sheehy writes in her 1991 bestseller *The Silent Passage*, "In trying to learn or talk about menopause, I found myself up against a powerful and mysterious taboo. My friends were adrift in the same fog of inexcusable ignorance. We couldn't help each other because none of us knew enough."[1] I think Ms. Sheehy would agree that "you have come a long way baby" since then.

Now women march in the street "taking back" their menopause. (I never knew anyone took it away.) They proudly proclaim the sisterhood of aging as a dominant social force, which it has become. I caution you not to fall prey to the "spiritual feminism" that pervades some of this literature. The pendulum of awareness has swung so far that several women have told me that they feel guilty for not having menopausal problems! Their point is that with this awareness explosion a wealth of negativism is infecting the common perception of menopause. This is a monumental problem, as the dominant attitude in this culture is both overtly or covertly one of considering menopause to be a disease. The medical profession is guilty of perpetuating this myth. A recent article in the medical journal *Menopause* concludes, "Clinical depression has become an endemic part of the female experience resulting in increased rates of medical service use, increased health care expenditure, and a lifetime risk of suicide as high as 15 percent."[2]

When menopause is discussed among friends or in the media, it is often presented in a less than attractive manner. It is much more sensational to talk about hardships and bad times than it is to talk of joy, celebrations, and solutions. I imagine it is similar to the way a woman's labor is talked about in the beauty shops and corporate boardrooms. Inevitably the discussion is energized by the details of a seventy-two-hour descent into hell orchestrated by a nine-pound alien who was happy in his little belly hot tub and resented being pulled through the drain! This is not to belittle those who truly had difficult labors, but the stories become embellished over time. You hear these stories because they are more interesting and dramatic. With time you begin to unconsciously view labor as this terrific ordeal because you have been continually bombarded with tales of terror. Menopause, now that it is talked about, has become like this.

You don't hear the great success stories. You don't hear about the huge number of women who have no complaints. You only read and hear the tragedies and tribulations of those who struggle with the menopause madness . . . over and over and over. So as time passes and God grants you a midlife, all of these images come racing back. If the war stories are from an important woman in your life, the negative impact can be immense. The increase in the visibility and discussion of menopause is generally very good, but be wary of the doomsayers.

Resources

Books abound on the subject. I have listed in the bibliography a few of my favorites. The Internet, that hotbed of accurate and timely knowledge on the level of the *Enquirer*, has hundreds of sites focusing exclusively on menopause and menopausal issues. The information superhighway is a good thing, but just as you wouldn't stop along the regular highway and pick up a dead skunk, so I caution you not to pick up every bit of information you find on the Internet. In all honesty, some of it stinks worse than a skunk. Table 1 lists some great Internet sites that provide useful and valid information. View all resources with a critical eye. Consider the source. Is there an agenda? Is there some hidden purpose in what you see and hear?

The Selling of Menopause

Menopause has become the latest darling of Madison Avenue. It has not only come out of the closet, but it has leaped into the bank vault. Why? Because there is a great deal of money to be made. With the aging of the baby boomers, more women are now entering meno-

Table 1
Internet Sites

www.holyhormones.md (your obvious first stop!)
www.menopause.org (website of North American Menopause Society, a great starting place)
www.herbs.org (excellent information and current research on herbal medicines)
www.healthywomen.org (good starting point for general health issues for women)
www.nof.org (home of the National Osteoporosis Foundation)
www.odyssee.net/~janine (A Friend Indeed, the oldest consumer-related menopause newsletter)
www.menopause-online.com (a balanced view of both traditional and nontraditional approaches)
www.dearest.com (Power Surge newsletter, excellent page, lots of wellpresented practical information)
www.bodywise.net (general health topics for the whole family)
www.acog.org (American College of Obstetricians and Gynecologists)
www.mediconsult.com (huge amount of information on any health re-lated topic, good discussions on menopause)
www.aimnet.com/~hyperion/meno/menotimes.index.html (Menotimes newsletter dedicated to alternative choices for dealing with menopause and osteoporosis)
www.christianity.net (a comprehensive clearinghouse for Christian websites, a must visit!)
www.healthy.net (good mix of traditional and nontraditional informa-tion on a variety of subjects)
www.csranet.com/~wes (my practice's webpage)

pause than in any other time in history. Women over sixty-five will be one of the fastest growing segments of the population. This is a huge market, as many drug company executives are discovering. In 1997 it is estimated that 83 million Americans spent over 27 billion dollars on alternative health care.[3] Much of this cash flowed for the purchase of herbs and vitamins, which are an important component of alternative approaches to menopause.

The pharmaceutical industry, in this country alone, is a multibillion-dollar industry. They have targeted this huge market of nonprescription medicines. The marketing approach to these substances, because they occur in nature and can't be patented, will be one of direct-to-consumer advertising. This approach will largely rely on name-brand loyalty and confidence to sell their product. Already pharmaceutical giants promote "menopause relief formulas" and "female remedies." There is some benefit from this increased attention to natural medicines in that it will inevitably spawn additional research in the United States, investigating efficacy and safety. My fear is that the poor quality and unpredictable reliability of products from unregulated manufacturers will throw a veil of impropriety over the entire industry. Thus natural medicine manufacturers must police their own to guarantee quality and consistency in their products, or the consumer will shun their inventories.

Menopause has become an industry. One of the most prescribed drugs in the past decade is Premarin, an estrogen replacement tablet. Menopause is a multifaceted economic diamond ready to be mined. The expansive market base that is largely untapped (remember only 17 percent of eligible women take hormone replacement therapy, or HRT) is being courted along with the even larger group of women who are looking for alternative approaches. I can see the future, and it is a Menopause Barbie!

Pick up any "woman's magazine" and you will be accosted with ads for hormone replacement therapy. If the publication's demographics are targeted to the over-thirty-five-age woman, I guarantee at least one ad will appear, possibly more. Notice the subtle nature of the ads. Almost all appeal to the vanity of their target audience. They scream: "Look good, feel good, and stay sexy!" Ads may not state it overtly; however, if you dissect the intent and presentation, they inevitably make direct or indirect reference to physical appearance, mental functioning, or sexuality. This is not by accident but by design.

Hormone replacement was originally promoted years ago as a cosmetic. It was a way to keep you "feminine forever." That attitude has persisted in Madison Avenue workrooms. It is this desire to stay young and thwart aging that will sell their products. Granted, they also emphasize the long-term benefits such as osteoporosis prevention, yet the subliminal message is "use hormones and stay beautiful." Focus groups and surveys reinforce that this message will sell their product.

The direct-to-consumer advertising for prescription drugs is a relatively new phenomenon. It is reminiscent of the snake oil salesman of the past who hawked elixir from the wagon direct to the eager townspeople. In the past these promotions for prescription drugs appeared only in medical and trade journals and relied on clinical information and data to sell their products. The target audience was the doctor; that was their customer.

With the explosion of popular interest in menopause, the drug companies have shifted their advertising strategy to focus on the consumer. The companies understand the current lack of information for the consumer, and they want to fill that gap. Needless to say they want to fill it with information that promotes their products. This is only good business, right? But is it good for the consumer?

The moral is: be critical of the information you receive. Evaluate the source. I am by no means suggesting that all information disseminated by drug manufacturers is suspect. Some generic facts and figures are helpful. However, they are in the business of selling, and any information they distribute will be designed to sell their products.

This marketing of menopause also reflects the differences in how a doctor and patient may view this transition. A woman is most likely to view menopause as a time of symptoms and changes that need attention, and her interest and actions are more reactive to these symptoms. Many physicians, on the other hand, continue to approach menopause as an estrogen-deficiency disease and prescribe hormones primarily for overall health benefits. Symptomatic treatment is a secondary gain. Menopause is no more an estrogen-deficiency disease than a headache is a Tylenol-deficiency disease! There are those in the medical community that feel strongly that every woman, with few exceptions, should be prescribed hormones!

I do not ascribe to that philosophy. I don't believe God created woman imperfectly with a built-in obsolescence. I don't feel that a woman was designed to automatically "lose her worth" at age fifty-one, as some would have you think. This "biomedical" view of menopause as a disease has galvanized the marketing of menopause. It is what drives the economic menopause machine. If the public recognizes this transition as a medical affliction then it only makes sense that it must be treated. And how do we do that in this country? Drugs! As more and more women are clamoring for other approaches, the slick marketers are saying, "Sure we have herbs and vitamins, take those (made by us) if you don't like our estrogen products." They are still perpetuating the myth of "menopause as a disease."

Many of the advertisements for estrogen, and much of the lay literature, covertly project the concept that if you don't use estrogen you will pitifully and inevitably end up as a wrinkled, sexless, old hag. This is not only untrue, but it is also an insult to women. You can live a vibrant, healthy, long life using a variety of techniques, foods, activities, and medicines if you so choose. The use of hormones is not the criteria for health, longevity, or physical beauty.

Many physicians and health care personnel are becoming more supportive of the concept of a "transitional" approach to menopause, an approach that is cognizant of the normalcy of the change and recognizes the importance of choice and responsibility.

THE FOUR A'S

Many of the lifestyle choices you make, such as diet and exercise, can dramatically affect your menopausal experience. Proverbs gives us other admonitions about the latter years, such as "Wisdom will multiply your days and add years to your life," and "Fear of the LORD lengthens one's life, but the years of the wicked are cut short."(Proverbs 10:27) We are meant to live a happy, long life, and for most women that means a third of it will be lived in the postmenopausal time. It is not a time to be complacent or anxious. It is a time, a season, to rejoice and celebrate what God has provided. The pages that follow give practical suggestions on how to do just that.

What is the prescription for midlife miracles? The four A's: attitude, action, aptitude, and apothecary.

Attitude

What we believe is our reality, what we *know* is our truth. "You will know the truth and the truth will set you free."(John 8:32) Believe in the celebration of menopause. Be glad for midlife. Your other options are not that great.

Action

There are two levels of action involved. First, act on what you know. The key to any person's success, whether in business or in the home, is taking action. A great idea is only great if acted upon. "So you see, it isn't enough just to have faith. Faith that doesn't show itself by good deeds is no faith at all—it is dead and useless." (James 2:17) If you do what you have always done you will get what you have always gotten. There is nothing sadder than a good idea that dies from loneliness or lack of attention. Whether that's using hormones, herbs, or massage therapy, whatever path God leads you to is the right one for you. "Your word is a lamp for my feet and a light for my path" (Ps.119:105).

Second, get off your behind and get moving! Exercise is the fountain of youth and a cleansing activity for mind and body. "Physical exercise has some value, but spiritual exercise is much more important, for it promises a reward in both this life and the next" (1 Tim. 4:8).

Aptitude

Educate yourself; learn your options. Ask questions, talk to others, and take responsibility. "Fear of the LORD is the beginning of knowledge. Only fools despise wisdom and discipline" (Proverbs 1:7).

Apothecary

Some of you may remember the old drugstores. Not only did they sell prescription medicines, but they had a lunch counter, a place where you could get the best herbs, and often a pharmacist who would jump at the chance to give you an opinion . . . about anything! The idea of foods and herbs as medicines will be explored (as will the other A's) in the following chapters.

Definitions

Before we go further, let's define some important terms so we all are thinking alike. (That's a scary thought, all of us thinking alike!)

Menopause is simply a stop in the periods. That's it. And this can only be identified in retrospect. In other words, a woman doesn't know it was her last period until six months have gone by and she has had no others.

Surgical menopause is when a woman's ovaries are removed prior to the time that they would normally cease functioning. This is most commonly done at the time of a hysterectomy; however, the ovaries are not removed automatically at every hysterectomy. A hysterectomy removes only the uterus and cervix. The uterus doesn't have a hormonal production role as do the ovaries, so simply removing the uterus does not cause surgical menopause even though the periods cease. If a woman has a hysterectomy *and* removal of her ovaries at age thirty-four, then she is surgically menopausal.

Don't be confused by the often-used terminology, *total hysterectomy* or *partial hysterectomy*. When people use these terms they are labeling a total hysterectomy as one in which the ovaries are removed, and a partial hysterectomy as one in which the ovaries remain. I make this distinction because of confusion that surrounds these terms. It is the removal of the ovaries that creates surgical menopause. Simply removing the uterus (the partial hysterectomy in slang terms) will not create a surgically menopausal woman since her ovaries are intact and still going full blast. It is the ovaries that are responsible for the hormone production, not the uterus. The average age for natural menopause is fifty-one.

Perimenopause is a more useful term in assessing symptoms. This is the time frame around the menopause. It can vary in its length and onset and is actually defined by the presence of symptoms. There is no set age or time that marks the perimenopause. It is as individual as your own experience. In other words, if you are forty-two and having severe hormonal hot flashes you can be considered to be in the perimenopause. Many women have no symptoms or warnings before their periods cease. For these women the only perimenopause is the time immediately after their periods cease. My mother is such a soul. To this day she can't understand what all this uproar over menopause is all about. She had (and still has) absolutely no symptoms! Nothing. *Nada.* She would rather I devote myself to real problems like remembering her birthday and calling on Sundays!

I use the term *postmenopausal* to describe the time after the periods cease. Many will continue to use perimenopausal to refer to this time, but I find that confuses people. Simply stated, perimenopause is the time leading up to menopause and postmenopause is the time after the cessation of menses. I am essentially using perimenopause and premenopause interchangeably.

PMS, or *premenstrual syndrome*, will be addressed with exuberance in the following chapter; however, it is important to state at the outset that this is a real problem. It is not imagined, and it is completely unacceptable to patronize a woman by saying, "Oh darling, it's only your hormones." It is a clinically identifiable syndrome with a physiological basis. The significance for the woman in midlife is that PMS symptoms may appear for the first time, and often PMS and perimenopausal symptoms are confused. Telling a woman in the throes of PMS that she is just experiencing a few hormonal fluctuations is like calling a hurricane a breath of fresh air. I take it seriously, and so should you. More on this later.

Estrogen is the predominant female hormone. In the female it can take several different chemical forms. It is the most abundant hormone of the triad that affects women and their cycles. The other two major hormones are progesterone and testosterone. Testosterone is commonly referred to as the "male hormone" largely because it is the hormone that does predominate in the male system. It is produced by the female in lower concentrations arid plays an important role in sexuality and well-being.

Another term you may hear is *climacteric*. This refers to the time around the menopause, and many equate this term with the perimenopause. I use it when I want to include both pre- and postmenopausal scenarios.

SUMMARY

Menopause is a normal natural transition in a woman's life. It is part of the grand plan from God and is not meant to be a time of worry and ill health. Current Western culture presents menopause as a declining, nonproductive, and negative time. This is not only false but also in direct conflict with what is stated in the Bible about aging. One's attitude toward midlife and menopause largely determines one's experience. God has a plan about how to make this transition a celebration, and, as believers, we must learn how this applies to us and our situations. Once you have the knowledge, it is critical that you take the next step, that of acting on that knowledge. This allows you to reap the fruit of your faith and beliefs. The four A's (Attitude, Action, Aptitude, and Apothecary) will serve as guideposts directing your journey. God designed woman to have a productive midlife and beyond, so full speed ahead!

ACTION CHALLENGE

Starting today shift your focus from one of worry and lack to one of praise and abundance. God has a plan and, no matter how old, how sick, how crabby, or how stubborn you are, that plan can be realized. The fulfillment of that plan depends solely on two forces, you and God. My money says God will do His part; your challenge is to do yours. Start today by making the decision to think differently.

CHAPTER TWO

Nature, Alternative Medicine, and the Bible

Sue Ellen was confused physically and spiritually. She was a bright, articulate mother of two who was struggling with her emotions and her body. She came to my office on a Friday afternoon complaining mainly of fatigue. "I'm always so tired, and I mean all the time! I sleep well at night, but by midday I am just dragging. Dr. Eaker, I'm too young to be this old!"

We talked about her physical symptoms, and then I did a good physical exam. As we talked it became apparent that she had read some books on herbs and energy (she was a take-charge person) but was bothered by the "philosophy" that seemed to pervade what she read. She didn't want to "take medicine" to improve her energy level, so she sought more natural approaches. She was a strong Christian, yet she was confused by what she was reading. "I have to wade through a lot of New Age mumbo jumbo to get to the information on alternative approaches that I want. Is this OK, or should I avoid this kind of stuff all together?"

Sue Ellen is not alone in her confusion. Is alternative medicine "unchristian"? Can a woman use herbs and vitamins and not compromise her religious beliefs? The answer to these and other questions depends on an accurate understanding of the terms. Along with a meteoric rise in interest in menopause has come resurgence in "natural" and "alternative" approaches to midlife and its changes. It is important to define these terms to avoid misunderstandings. Don't be like the ninety-eight-year-old man who went to his doctor for a checkup and left after being told he was in excellent health for his age, except for a slight hearing loss. The doctor saw him on the street the next day arm in arm with a beautiful young lady and asked him incredulously, "What are you doing?"

The old fella replied, "Doc, yesterday you told me to get a hot mamma and be cheerful!"

The doctor shook his head and cried, "No, I said you have a heart murmur so be careful!"

It is easy to "mis-hear" when ambiguous and unclear terms are used. Medicine is buried in jargon, and one of the biggest complaints that patients voice is that the health care professional talks in "medical speak."

Let me attempt to translate the "medical speak" into "normal speak." I consider a "natural" substance anything that occurs *by design* in nature or in a healthy body. Therefore, it does not include synthetic chemicals or medications. For purposes of this discussion anything that is not a naturally occurring substance is not considered "natural."

For example, progesterone cream contains the exact chemical substance that is in a woman's body. This is a "natural" substance. Even though the actual product is made in a laboratory through a process of chemical reactions, the final substance is one that is "naturally" occurring in the healthy human. Conversely, Provera, or medroxyprogesterone acetate, is a substance created in the lab to facilitate its oral use. This is not a "natural" substance. Nowhere in the human will you find a molecule of medroxyprogesterone acetate. Nowhere in nature will you find medroxyprogesterone acetate, or norethindrone, or other progesterone-like drugs. Those substances are progestigens and are used in hormone replacement therapy; however, their effects can be vastly different than those of progesterone. I will explore this difference in much greater detail later.

Don't Worry. Be Happy!

This definition of *natural* is extremely inclusive. This implies nothing about effectiveness, side effects, or cost. It also does not imply who can or who cannot utilize or recommend such substances. Psalm 24:1 says, "The Earth is the Lord's and everything in it." There is an innate obligation and responsibility to understand and explore what God has provided. God knows our needs and provides for them through a variety of channels. Jesus said, "Your heavenly Father already knows all your needs, and he will give you all you need from day to day if you live for him and make the Kingdom of God your primary concern. So don't worry about tomorrow, for tomorrow will bring its own worries. Today's trouble is enough for today." (Matthew 6:34)

Substances should not be universally acknowledged as healthy by virtue of their "natural" label. I was at the beach one summer, and my wife asked me to take a picture of our two little girls (then five and three) for a Christmas card. We wandered through the sand dunes until we found a beautiful display of flowers, sand, and surf that would appropriately highlight my little angels. They picked a couple of the pretty flowers (at my request) to hold to attempt to emulate the pictures I had seen from much more qualified photographers.

After I had taken what I was sure was a Pulitzer prize photo, a couple on the beach casually commented that the pretty flowers that our girls were holding were an extremely poisonous variety that would be very harmful if gnawed on by our young models! Needless to say I quickly snatched the flowers from their hands, and as they cried I tried to explain to them why the pretty flowers were not good to play with. To this day my daughter delights in telling company about the time Daddy tried to poison her! My point is that just because something is labeled as "natural" doesn't mean that it is necessarily healthy or useful. Not all of God's creation was meant to be appreciated in the same way!

A common misperception about "natural" products is that they have few side effects. Many herbal preparations, when ingested in improper amounts, may produce marked complications. An example is the herb Mu Haung that is in a lot of the "natural" weight loss products. This herb has been associated with heart arrhythmia (irregular heartbeats). Another example involves the fat-soluble vitamins A, D, E, and K, which can build up to toxic levels if taken in high enough doses over an extended time. You can get too much of a good thing. Combining some "natural" substances can also be harmful. Their side effects can be synergistic and counterproductive.

An issue rapidly coming to the forefront is the combination of prescription medicines and herbal treatments. One survey stated that over 15 million people combined one or more medications with one or more herbal products. This same survey asserted that about 60 percent of people using herbal products don't discuss them with their health care professionals. This is of great concern because there are some combinations that can be dangerous.

As you explore your options, part of the educational challenge is to share them with your doctor or pharmacist. Keep an accurate and current list of all prescription medications, and don't be hesitant to discuss your use of alternative therapies with your doctor. On more than one occasion I have asked a patient whether they take any medicines on a regular basis. The response was negative, until with further questioning I discovered they have a drawer full of vitamins, herbs, and supplements. I now am more specific in my questioning and purposely query about nonprescription drug use.

If your doctor is not receptive to your inquiries and information on this topic, find another doctor. A healthy balance requires initiating a dialogue with your doctor about any possible drug interactions. Thankfully, there is a great margin of safety with most "natural" products; however, be smart. Using "natural" substances is not an excuse to put your brain on a shelf.

No Quick Fix

Many of my patients tell me that using herbs and vitamins can be quite challenging. Sorting through the hundreds of brands and dosages and staying on a consistent regimen takes effort. If women are looking for a quick, easy fix to their symptoms, they will be disappointed, because a long-term successful regimen, whether hormone replacement therapy or "the naturals," involves commitment and persistence. Clearly, the message is that there is no panacea. God has provided many wonderful herbs, foods, and drinks that can markedly benefit every woman in midlife. You must learn to use them wisely and in the manner that the Creator intended. I will revisit this in greater detail later.

What do I mean when I refer to "alternative" medicine? Many women have a preconceived idea of what that term means. In other words, they know what it means cognitively, but there is inevitably an emotional rider to this understanding. I challenge you to view this with an open mind and heart. Don't let prior beliefs be impediments to understanding legitimate choices and options.

I remember the story of a young woman who was absolutely convinced that she was dead. She was, in reality, very much alive and her frustrated family finally employed the services of a local psychiatrist to help her. After spending several nonproductive sessions with the woman trying to convince her that she was not dead, he resorted to a logical approach. He brought down one of his anatomy books and painstakingly walked her through the functioning of the circulatory system. They finally agreed that dead people don't bleed. The psychiatrist then took a lance and pricked the girl's finger and drew a drop of blood. Proudly he looked at her and said, "Now what does that tell you?"

The girl excitedly exclaimed, "Oh my! Dead people do bleed!" She was obviously stuck in a frame of mind that wouldn't allow her to see beyond her sphere of reference.

Most people view "alternative" approaches as any therapy outside the mainstream of current medically-accepted treatment and diagnostic modalities. During a discussion with a refined older lady about alternative methods of dealing with menopausal complaints, I noticed a look of apprehension on her face. When I commented on this, she blurted out, "You're not going to get naked and burn incense are you?" Images of crystals and Eastern mystics cloud the perception of what I consider alternative.

Alternative Approaches

The definition of *alternative* is totally dependent on the era and culture in which it is used. Currently acceptable medical treatment is defined by the governing bodies of national associations and by the local laws and customs where it is practiced. To the Navajo child, raised on a reservation in Arizona, the juice of the cactus may be an acceptable traditional treatment for ulcers; whereas, the prescription drug Ranitidine may be viewed as "alternative." So traditional and nontraditional medical practices are culturally dependent. They can and do change with time.

Many thought Edward Jenner was insane when he proposed preventing smallpox by injecting a similar virus from cows into humans. There were cartoons that depicted women receiving the smallpox vaccine and watching in horror as a cow head or udder sprouted from their necks; however, Jenner's proposal set the stage for modern immunizations!

What is once thought of as state-of-the-art may at a latter date be viewed as archaic, and the reverse is true. However, there are some universal and constant truths. What the Bible says about health and long life is still applicable today! It is as valid now as it was two centuries ago. This testifies to the eternal truths that the Bible teaches. Because God is living, eternal, and unchanging, you can trust Him to help His people in this generation, just as He helped in past generations.

Complementary Medicine

I actually prefer the term *complementary* medicine instead of "alternative." The connotation is that this is a different approach than the traditional; however, the two can be simultaneously employed. "Alternative" implies exclusivity whereas "complementary" implies inclusiveness, and that is more consistent with my belief system. The term *alternative medicine* is unfortunately fused to a particular philosophical and pseudo-spiritual movement. The New Age movement has been identified with some alternative medical practices because of a few shared methodologies and beliefs. This is derived from the similarities and shared vocabulary of herbalism, visualization, and meditation with Eastern religions and philosophies. In reality these associations are invalid, although it is incumbent on the individual to separate the "spiritual" foundation from the scientific validity. It is wrong to issue a blanket condemnation of alternative therapies based on incorrect and ignorant associations.

I don't like the term "New Age" because I don't know how to define it. It brings about an emotional response that is fraught with misunderstanding. To many Christians the New Age is a major affront to their beliefs, and I agree with their apprehension, based on my own interpretation of what "New Age" means. However, there is little new in the "New Age," and I don't see this as a major problem in the areas we will be discussing. Nevertheless I will choose to refer to less traditional approaches as complementary treatments throughout the rest of this book. I will also attempt to distinguish between the methods and the philosophy when appropriate.

The Bible as a User's Manual

What does the Bible say about designs for living, and how does this apply to midlife and menopause? Both the Old and New Testaments contain specific and practical guidance on foods, moods, exercise, prayer, stress, anxiety, herbs, attitude, and healing. The Bible not only gives guidelines to emulate, it also gives specific examples and role models.

The women of the Bible serve as role models for today's woman. Virginia Owens, in her book *Daughters of Eve*, asks,

> How much has life really changed for women? Are there, in fact, gendered propensities that persist over time, threads that run through time and across cultures revealing essential patterns? Are we, even after centuries of change, still "sisters under the skin" with the Middle Eastern, North African, and Mediterranean women who span the biblical pages? Do their fears and sorrows,

> hopes and joys connect with ours? If we paid attention to them, would they have anything significant to say to us?[1]

She then proceeds to answer those penetrating and relevant questions with a resounding "yes" by showing in excellent detail how women in the Bible speak clearly and loudly to the women of today. Such unforgettable personalities as Ruth, Naomi, Mary, Martha, and Hannah provide excellent examples of God's guidance on living, acting, and believing.

It is a logical assessment that the greatest "how to" book ever written provides a plethora of practical mentors, and I will use some of these women's stories to illustrate Gods' plan for a successful journey through menopause.

Menopause Is a Season

> There is a time for everything,
> A season for every activity under heaven.
> A time to be born and a time to die.
> A time to plant and a time to harvest.
> A time to kill and a time to heal.
> A time to tear down and a time to rebuild.
> A time to cry and a time to laugh.
> A time to grieve and a time to dance.
> A time to scatter stones and a time to gather stones.
> A time to embrace and a time to turn away.
> A time to search and a time to lose.
> A time to keep and a time to throw away.
> A time to tear and a time to mend.
> A time to be quiet and a time to speak up.
> A time to love and a time to hate.
> A time for war and a time for peace. (Eccl. 3:1–8)

This familiar passage illustrates that just as there is a time for living and loving, building and tearing down, so there is a time for life changes.

Menopause and Old Age

Menopause is the end of reproduction but not the end of production. Many of the negative feelings in the Western world toward menopause arise from its close association with aging. At my seminars around the country I always ask the audience to play the "free association" game. When I say the word menopause inevitably someone will yell out "old" or "aging," and it gets worse from there.

Whether we like it or not, this is still a youth-oriented culture. Mirroring modern culture, the advertisement industry reflects the desirability of youth. Conversely, aging is portrayed as that horrid condition to be avoided at all cost. You may think this is an exaggeration, yet look closely at magazine ads or TV commercials. This obsession with being or looking young is evident.

Some will resort to ridiculous gyrations to retain at least the physical appearance of youth. The gross misperception is that a physical change will be translated into an emotional transformation: If we look young, we will feel young. Those who have attempted to keep pace with a granddaughter on a mall outing realize that looking young and feeling young are not always compatible. No matter how young we think we are, physical laws dictate that there comes a time when our knees buckle but our belts won't. Some say you have reached that mature age when your back goes out more than you do. For those who are feeling a bit dismayed at this reality, remember the words of the Almighty as written in Isaiah: "I will be your God throughout your lifetime—until your hair is white with age. I made you, and I will care for you. I will carry you along and save you." (Isaiah 46:4)

Samuel Johnson wrote, "He that would pass the latter part of his life with honor and decency, must, when he is young, consider that he shall one day be old; and remember, when he is old, that he has once been young."

The Youthful Look

We are the most nipped, tucked, scraped, and sucked generation ever. Dr. Sara Murray Jordan says, "A much more effective and lasting method of facelifting than surgical technique is happy thinking, new interests, and outdoor exercise."

Ecclesiastes puts this in perspective when it reads, "Don't let the excitement of youth cause you to forget your Creator. Honor him in your youth before you grow old and no longer enjoy living."(Ecclesiastes12:1) I would argue against the concept that just becoming old interferes with your enjoyment of life, yet the point here is to live in the present.

Why would so many risk the complications and the discomforts of surgery to achieve the young look? Vanity and the desire to counteract the physical aging process are common reasons. Solomon gives us sage advice in Proverbs 31:30: "Charm is deceptive, and beauty does not last; but a woman who fears the LORD will be greatly praised. Reward her for all she has done. Let her deeds publicly declare her praise."

The obsession with youthful looks is like a Band-Aid on a gaping sore. It covers the external evidence of hurt and pain, yet the wound still exists. The unfortunate perception is that by changing the outer surface you change the truth of who you are. All of this is an illusion. The reality is that plastic surgery is altering the cover; it has no effect on the actual aging process. It doesn't change the basic biochemistry of cellular aging. In many ways it's like the banana with the beautiful enticing yellow peel that quickly turns your stomach when you take away the peel to reveal a bruised and browned inner core. If people were truly interested in slowing the aging process, they would put their time and energy into things such as exercise, proper diet, minimizing sun exposure, and taking proper antioxidant supplements.

One of the most bizarre and contradictory activities of our quick-fix culture is suntanning. Our present society perceives a bronze tan on light skin as a sign of health and youthfulness, while the reality is just the opposite. There is no other single endeavor that promotes an aging appearance more rapidly than extended sun exposure. It is ironic that the desire to achieve a youthful healthy look actually does just the opposite. This is intrinsic to the cultural dislike for delayed gratification. People want the immediate gratification of the suntanned look, yet they don't consider the long-term consequences. How many times in daily life are long-term benefits sacrificed for the short-term gains? We want it yesterday. Delayed gratification has become synonymous with no gratification. The problem in midlife and menopause is that the invoices from our youth come due at this time.

Don't Be a Victim

What we believe becomes our reality, so it is understandable that menopause has developed a negative aura in Western society. It is not that way in other cultures. Social anthropologists find that negative symptoms of menopause are almost nonexistent in cultures where aging is revered and respected! The word for "hot flash" doesn't even exist in Japan. A study done a few years ago compared the symptoms of menopause cross-culturally and found that the single greatest factor that influenced the intensity and variety of symptoms of menopause was the individual's perception of aging! This is exciting information in that it shifts responsibility from the external to the internal. In other words, menopause doesn't have to be something that happens to you, it is something you can influence. Instead of simply reacting to symptoms, you can train your mind and body to not ever experience any symptoms!

A woman can have a marked impact on her menopausal experience by changing her thoughts. You can go from a victim mentality to a belief system that promotes control over your physical and emotional destiny. This is a revelation to many women who have been inundated with messages that this thing called menopause was inevitably bad, and worse, that women were powerless to do anything about it. There is control; there are choices. You can look to Scripture for encouragement and advice, you can pray for divine guidance, you can change the way you think about menopause, and you can take action to make this a reality.

This time in your life is a joyous one and can be celebrated.

Integration

If there is something unhealthy or troublesome in your thoughts, it cannot help but impact your physical body. We have all experienced situations where our thoughts and emotions were the direct precursors to physical symptoms. A classic example of this type of interaction is the panic attack. If you have never experienced this phenomenon, it is hard to describe the intensity of both the physical and emotional feelings. It often begins as a rapid heart rate and difficulty breathing and is followed by a profound sense of dread and fear of dying. This in turn leads to a heightened "fight or flight" response and can ultimately result in severe hyperventilation and physical and emotional collapse. The physical symptoms are secondary to anxiety and chemical changes in the brain. In turn, much of the anxiety is in direct response to the physical symptoms. These two responses feed on each other and the cycle perpetuates until one or both systems collapse.

A similar chain of events can occur if one's spiritual life is not in harmony. It sets up a tension that can be manifested in physical and emotional symptoms. Just as a rubber band can only be stretched so far before it breaks, so this inner turmoil can progress only so far before the tension is released, often in the form of physical or emotional symptoms.

There is a fascinating branch of science called psychoneuroimmunology that studies the effects of thoughts, feelings, and emotions on the immune system. In this age of AIDS awareness, much is known about the importance of a properly functioning immune system. This area of study has shown conclusively that strong emotional states can have a profound influence on how, for example, white blood cells produce antibodies that fight disease. Being anxious or upset can lead to physical illness! Anger has been shown to impede the white blood cell's ability to ward off invading viruses. This may explain why colds and runny noses proliferate during times of high stress. In his book *Health and Medicine in the Methodist Tradition*, E. Brooks Holifield writes, "A diseased brain could produce delirium of spirit, disordered nerves could engender distempered thoughts, and obstructed circulation could create spiritual temptations."[2]

This miraculous interdependence serves as a natural guardian of health. Conversely, it can also serve as a source of multiple stresses and imbalances. All menopausal experiences have an impact on not just your physical body but your emotions, thoughts, and feelings, as well as your walk with God.

God's Plan

God wants us to be healthy. He cares for our natural bodies. God wants us to use common sense *and* medical science to achieve a balance in mind, soul, and body. But just as menopause is a unique experience for every woman, so the way God guides you toward health may be different. God may lead you to certain foods or exercises that are tremendously effective for treating a specific problem, yet those same choices may be ineffective or even harmful for another person. The challenge is to take the knowledge available to you and prayerfully consider its application to your situation. God will not let you down. He designed us to be healthy vibrant beings, and doesn't leave us without the provisions to achieve this optimal balance of mind, body, and spirit. Patch Adams, a well-known physician and clown, says health is a happy, vibrant life, doing the most with what you have, joyously.

Why is it important that you take care of your body and its needs? Should you assume that God will provide the needed healing for all of your ills or symptoms? Is it right to use medical science in helping with your maladies? Look at 1 Corinthians 6:19–20: "Don't you know that your body is the temple of the Holy Spirit, who lives in you and was given to you by God? You do not belong to yourself, for God bought you with a high price. So you must honor God with your body." This does not say it just would be nice to promote a healthy body; it is a command to honor God with your body. It doesn't say it would be really neat if you took care of yourself. It says you *must* honor God with your body. The implied message is that to let your body fall into disrepair is to dishonor its Creator. You *must* honor God by how you take care of your body.

God always provides the mechanisms to fulfill His commands. This is consistent throughout the Bible. The choice is whether to act on these instructions or to ignore them. It is never too late to make that choice. I hear women remark daily that they have never exercised or have always eaten poorly or never took vitamins in the past, so why start now? Even more distressing are those who feel a sense of hopelessness because of previous failures at living a healthy lifestyle. The endless diets, the yearlong memberships in the gym that turn into two weeks of use, all contribute to this "What's the use?" mentality. These experiences definitely color your present behaviors, but God is an awesome God! With the proper motivation, education, and prayerful consideration of His desires for your health, any obstacle can be overcome.

I am not an impractical optimist. I do live in the real world and realize these changes are a major lifestyle shift for some. I understand that it is much easier to get your exercise from the channel changer than from the stationary bike. For some the only exertion you undertake is jumping to conclusions or running from the truth.

Gary Severson, writing in the *Christian Reader*, tells of an old guy who bragged to his preacher. "Yes, Pastor, everyday I get out of bed and run around the block six times!" The preacher was significantly impressed until the old fellow continued. "Then I shove the block back under the bed and lay back down!"

Achieving Wholeness

Remember, as followers of Jesus and believers of God's Word, we must tend to our bodies as well as our minds and spirits. We must honor God with our bodies, and we must use any means available to achieve health (wholeness). This may mean new and better dietary choices. This may mean starting an exercise program. This may mean using hormone replacement therapy or utilizing vitamins and dietary supplements. This may mean taking time to meditate or to pray to reduce stress. The possibilities are endless, and I will show you how to identify those practices that will be most helpful to you in the midlife. The goal is to care for your body, mind, and soul to the glory of God.

God designed us for a long and healthy life. He states that a long life is a result of proper choices and behavior. Psalm 91 says, "I will satisfy them with a long life and give them my salvation."

In Exodus 20:12 God states, "Honor your father and mother. Then you will live a long, full life in the land the LORD your God will give you."

Put out to Pasture

God intends for you to live a long life *when* you have faith and obedience to His Word. Do nonbelievers live long lives? Of course they do. The promise of a long life should not be viewed as a prize or reward for believing, but as a greater opportunity to fulfill your purpose. It is not so important how *long* we live as it is *how* we live. God did not create women with a planned obsolescence. I recently read an article in *Parade* magazine that absolutely horrified me. It was profiling an "anti-aging" doctor and he was quoted as saying, "Women were engineered to make lots of babies and then collapse at about age forty. They were not meant to endure the high stress of a career and postpone childbirth until their late thirties. Now that the average age span is almost 80, women need help to lead a modern life." This attitude contributes to the negative feelings that many women have about aging.

It is hard for me to believe that in God's perfect design He said that a woman will "collapse" at age forty. Some consumer products are designed to last a certain time and then break down. Vacuum cleaners, yes. Women, no. How many of us are struck by the apparent coincidence of the lawn mower exploding two days after the warranty expires? Am I being paranoid? Probably. But next time the TV tube goes out, check the date on your service contract!

Look at Proverbs 3:1–2: "My child, never forget the things I have taught you. Store my commands in your heart, for they will give you a long and satisfying life." It is important to notice that a long and satisfying life is not an automatic occurrence. The intentional will of God is that people remain healthy, but each of the verses is predicated on the concept that it is your choices that determine if you are going to reap the fruits of God's promises. This reinforces the idea that the blessings of along and healthy life are there for the taking, *yet you must do your part.* You have to make healthy lifestyle decisions. You cannot abdicate your responsibility for doing the right thing. Being a Christian demands that you be accountable for your health practices. Being a Christian does not mean putting your brain or body on "ignore."

Taking Responsibility

You are not left to struggle with this on your own. God has provided the road map, the guidebook, the ultimate training manual to help on this journey. There is a strong personal responsibility in making these choices. Much of the disease and poor health experienced today is generated from unhealthy lifestyle choices. If you analyze the leading causes of morbidity and mortality in the United States, you find many "lifestyle illnesses." Number one is heart disease, a condition that individuals can markedly affect by their actions and decisions. Your diet and activity level can have just as much impact on your risk factors for heart disease as your genes. Number two is cancer. The leading cause of cancer death in women is lung cancer. This is directly correlated to the increase in the number of women smoking.

God intends for you to be healthy. You were designed that way; however, you must take responsibility in using information, education, and action to facilitate this intrinsically healthy state. You cannot change the natural consequences of your actions. If you smoke, you dramatically increase your chances of lung cancer. God does not send lung cancer to you as punishment for smoking; it is the natural result of a conscious choice to abuse your body.

This concept of personal responsibility applies to menopausal changes. If you listen and obey God's words and take action to implement what you hear, you will find the fruits of your labors to be abundant.

Does this mean that as Christians you won't become ill? Of course not. Anyone who uses that argument is missing the point. Simply being a Christian does not exclude you from the sickness and mishaps of a world bound by natural laws and consequences. Bad things happen to good people. However, you can control a major portion of your health and wellness by wise choices.

You can also control your response to illness. In his book *Tuesdays with Morrie*, Mitch Albom writes about Morrie Shwartz, a favorite college mentor struck with Lou Gehrig's disease.

> What impressed me about Morrie was the honest acceptance of his illness and his exuberance to continue to live each day. He was reduced to total paralysis by this horrible disease yet his mind flourished and he cherished each day he was alive. Close to his death he said, "So many people walk around with a meaningless life. They seem half-asleep, even when they are busy doing things that seem important. This is because they are chasing the wrong things. The way you get meaning into your life is to devote yourself to loving others, devote yourself to the community around you, and devote yourself to creating something that give you purpose and meaning."[3]

When Mitch asked him about his disease, Morrie replied, "It's only horrible if you see it that way. It's horrible to watch my body slowly wilt away to nothing. But it is also wonderful because of all the time I get to say good-bye. Not everyone is so lucky!"[4]

Health is a harmony of mind, body, and spirit. You can be ill physically yet still be whole in mind and spirit. When one part of the healing triad is broken, the others can provide support for a while.

Running to Win

Menopause can be compared to a foot race. The apostle Paul was fond of this analogy. I am a runner (please, not a jogger!), so this comparison rings true for me. A marathon is a painful yet exhilarating experience. There is no escaping the conclusion that at some point in a 26.2 mile course you are going to feel pain. When I run a marathon, most of the time I am simply praying, "Lord give me this day my daily *breath*!" The question every marathon runner asks in every race is, "Do I have the will to go on?" Some of us pose that question earlier in the race than others, but even world-class runners at some point say to themselves, "Is it worth it?" Your approach to menopause and the years beyond is much like a marathon. You spend the first fifty or so years of life preparing for the event. You learn; you train; you experience life. All this follows you to the race. No one arrives at the start line without the sum of their previous life experience with them. Just as in a race, much of how you "perform" in the menopause is dependent on your preparation.

Most athletes will tell you that the training, the education, and the attitude going into the event are more important than the actual race. If you prepare properly, you have no fear. That is not to say the race will not be challenging, but because of your preparation, the apprehension will evaporate and you will face the struggle with a sense of joy and confidence. At this point the race becomes a celebration. If you prepare properly, in mind, body, and spirit, menopause will be a celebration.

Action Challenge

Find a good reference book on herbs and vitamins (I've listed several in the bibliography) and do some research. Educate yourself, and you will be surprised at how much more comfortable you feel with your options.

SECTION TWO

"I Thought I was Over This!" PMS and the Rest

CHAPTER THREE

The Who, What, and Why of PMS

Sandra (not her real name) was angry and upset. That was apparent as soon as she came into my office one fall afternoon. Her whole manner was tense.

"Dr. Eaker, I think I must be falling apart," she said, trying to hold back tears. "I don't know what is happening to me."

What was happening to her were changes that were affecting her family, her job, and her marriage. She was feeling helpless and frightened. Sandra revealed that over the past five to six months she had noticed that she had become quick to anger and yelled at the kids frequently in what she called "enthusiastic language."

"Yesterday, John, my six-year-old, said he wanted a Power Ranger figure for his next birthday. I said we would wait and see as it got closer to the day. Well, he kept on asking all through the day. You know how kids do? Not really meaning to irritate me. And normally it wouldn't have, but I finally just blew up. I yelled at him and told him to not say another word and even sent him to his room!

"A year ago I would have tolerated the constant request without much of a thought, but not any more. It is as if I couldn't help myself. I felt so out of control, it just wasn't me. And then I felt so bad afterwards, I thought, what will happen next? And these feelings affect Steve, my husband, also. He's a wonderful husband and a great father, but I swear there are times that I don't want him even to look at me. It's not that he does anything wrong, but when I'm in one of those 'moods.' he can't do anything right! He actually tells me that there is a look I have that means 'stay away,' and he has learned to do just that."

Sandra's work was also reflecting this change of moods and attitude. She was short with her clients and was not very accepting of her coworkers' simple mistakes. People were beginning to avoid her.

"There are times I feel pretty good, but there are times when I really don't like myself. And it's not all emotional changes," she said. "On some days I'm so bloated I feel like a blimp. I have this dull ache lower down like my period is about to start, but just can't begin. And worst of all, there are times when I could sit down and eat a whole cow if my family would let me. It's terribly frustrating to me because I have never been this way before. Oh sure, I used to get a little moody now and then, but it never amounted to anything. I'm afraid I am going to drive my kids away, lose my job, and shoot my husband!"

When Sandra confided her feelings to a few friends, they suggested that it might be her "hormones," and that's how she ended up in my office. After hearing her complaints I asked a few questions and began to get a clearer picture of Sandra's all-too-common problem. She had noticed that her moodiness and short temper followed a pattern. She could almost pinpoint the day in her cycle that the changes "come on me like a cloud." And they generally got better after her period, although sometimes the feelings persisted to a lesser degree all month. Her periods were still fairly regular; however, she had experienced intermittently what she thought were hot flashes. She was confused because some of her friends said it was the change of life, but she thought that only happened after her periods stopped. She also didn't think it was PMS because she had never been bothered by that before; and after all, wasn't she too old, at forty-two, to be having PMS?

After a good exam and a few additional inquiries, we decided on a few simple blood tests that would help in answering some of her questions. As it turned out, the blood work indicated that she was still ovulating and producing estrogen and progesterone, so she was not menopausal.

Is It PMS or Menopause?

Her history was characteristic of premenstrual syndrome as experienced in the midlife. In fact, Sandra's story is common today, but unfortunately doesn't often have a happy ending. Either the woman doesn't seek assistance, or when she does is misdiagnosed. Too many times the symptoms are ignored because of a woman's perception that she just has to live with it. There are many symptoms that have similar or overlapping causes, especially in perimenopausal women. It is vitally important to determine the true cause. PMS and perimenopause are related, yet they are two separate entities, and therefore the treatments are very different. Confusion often arises because the type and severity of symptoms can be similar in both PMS and the perimenopause, and they both occur commonly in a woman's early forties. I will show you how to make the distinction and diagnosis, and we will explore what the Bible says about PMS symptoms. (Yes, it does have a lot to say!) I will explain various treatment options and, more importantly, discuss who should and should not be treated.

PMS Defined

PMS is real. It is not in your head. It is not imagined. For years women have been maligned, ridiculed, and told, "It's just that time of the month." Whatever we (and by "we," I mean the predominantly male medical establishment) didn't understand was categorized as imaginary or unproven. There is no doubt medicine has come a long way in understanding the physiology of PMS, and has thus been able to better identify and treat this common problem. Approximately 90 percent of women having periods experience some premenstrual symptoms. Like menopause, it is individualized. In my practice I have seen everything from mild cramping to full psychotic breakdowns. The symptoms can be physical, emotional, or a combination of the two. There is no "classic" PMS. There may be certain similarities in symptoms, yet the experience is unique for everyone.

Premenstrual syndrome is defined as a *recurrent*, *predictable*, and *bothersome* group of symptoms that affects a woman physically and/or mentally. These symptoms can be mild or severe; they can be single or multiple. The medical profession is currently debating the semantics of PMS, using such terms as *premenstrual dysphoric disorder* and *premenstrual magnification syndrome*. These distinctions are helpful in clinical research, as they give a consistency and validity to the study of this entity. However, to Sally Mae on Main Street, USA, they don't mean much. For everyday folk, PMS is still the most useful term. This is what I will use throughout the book.

Let us look at the definition a little closer, because it is just as important to clarify what PMS is, as it is to know what it is not. Many women have incorrectly assumed that any physical or emotional aberration can be attributed to PMS. For some it has become a label for any change that takes place. This is wrong and potentially dangerous. Assuming all symptoms are due only to fluctuations in the hormonal cycle can miss other more serious problems. Be careful about wearing blinders when it comes to hormones. They can be the source of many symptoms, but so can many other entities. Hey, if it were easy you wouldn't be reading this now!

Know the Problem

The symptoms of PMS are ***recurrent***. They happen time and time again. The scientific community has chosen to make three months of recurrent symptoms the standard to define PMS. This allows women to make sure they are dealing with hormonally-based, repetitive symptoms and not an isolated event that may trigger symptoms once or twice.

For example, Susan had a terrible week at work. She was given a new batch of responsibilities and virtually no time to complete them. Her stress level was sky-high. Around the house she was short with the kids and snapped at her husband over almost any comment. Her period started, and she assumed that her unusual behavior was related. She thought, I know why I'm acting this way. It is my PMS talking, not me. What Susan didn't take into account was that she rarely had emotional changes around her period. It was unusual for her to even know when it was going to start. This recent behavioral change was more correctly attributed to stress and not PMS.

Is this so important? You bet it is! How these behavioral changes are perceived and the prospects of their continuation are intimately linked to correctly identifying the source. Also, any form of treatment would be based on the source of the symptoms and may vary accordingly. There is no question that stress and PMS can coexist. The reality is that most of the time they do. However, it is important to ascertain what is true PMS and what is stress-related. The key is sticking to the definition and making sure your symptoms meet those criteria. Stress and PMS can act as modifiers of each other's symptoms. If you are in a stressful situation, PMS symptoms will be magnified. Likewise, women who have bad PMS deal with stress differently during the luteal phase of the menstrual cycle as compared to other times.

There is a tremendous variety of symptoms associated with PMS. In true PMS the same symptoms generally repeat themselves, although a woman certainly can develop new or additional symptoms. For example, Sandra's symptoms of moodiness and short temper were repeated over and over each month. She did experience some bloating that developed later, yet it wasn't present from the start. Your life situation at any given time can impact the nature and intensity of symptoms, but the underlying consistency is still there.

The symptoms are ***predictable***. They are generally the same symptoms (they may vary in intensity), and they usually occur at the same time every cycle. The most common time for symptoms to arise is in the luteal phase of the menstrual cycle. Those are the days between ovulation and the onset of the period. In women who have a 28-32 day cycle, the luteal phase of the cycle is about days 14-28 (that is for all you obsessive counters).

A key part of this definition is that, for the majority of women, true PMS gets better with the onset of the period. I have women describe it as a physical and emotional feeling that all will be OK. It is as if they have been in a darkened room and suddenly someone comes in and pulls up the shades. They wake up and know they feel better.

If your symptoms persist after the period or continue into the first part of the cycle, you need to reassess whether you have PMS or some other disorder. Other conditions can cause the same symptoms, so it is vital to make the distinction. The biggest mistake made with PMS is labeling any unfavorable behavior as secondary to PMS. The PMS label has often been used as a scapegoat. There are exceptions to every rule; but, for most people, if this time frame of symptoms is not met, you need to entertain the idea that other things are occurring. A monumental mistake is approaching hormone disturbances with tunnel vision. Nothing can be viewed in isolation. If the classic symptom profile and timing is off, look elsewhere. It may still turn out to be PMS, but don't limit yourself by limiting your exploration.

Many thyroid disorders, metabolic diseases, clinical depressions, menopausal changes, and psychiatric disorders go undiagnosed or labeled as PMS. Here is where a competent, caring health care professional can act as a good resource. He or she can help in identifying other symptoms that may arise from these associated conditions and can suggest appropriate laboratory work that may diagnose a problem. For example, I will usually check a thyroid stimulating hormone level (TSH) to evaluate the function of the thyroid gland in most women for whom I am entertaining the diagnosis of PMS. Thyroid disease is so prevalent in women that I feel it is appropriate to evaluate in this situation.

There are many additional tests and evaluations that are available, and a good clinician can determine which would be appropriate based on your history. Table 2 lists some common medical conditions that can mimic PMS. There is no blood test that will diagnose PMS. That has to come from a close examination of your individual symptoms.

The symptoms are ***bothersome***. Just ask anyone who suffers from PMS, and you will quickly learn that it is not a walk in the park. "It is better to live alone in the desert than with a crabby, complaining wife" (Prov. 21:19).

This is an important component of the definition, because many times numerous symptoms may exist, yet they are of such minor consequence that they are not considered unusual or bothersome. Remember that the major reason to diagnose PMS is to treat its symptoms. I like this part of the definition because it places the responsibility for treatment where it belongs, with the patient. Ultimately you, and only you, can decide if the PMS problems you experience need treatment. This gives back the control to you, the one who is most affected by any decisions made. If you experience a few minor cramps, yet they are repetitive and predictable, do you have PMS? From a practical standpoint, no, because the symptoms have such a minor impact on your life that they don't warrant any treatment.

The key distinction is that these symptoms must be disturbing to the one experiencing them. It is not unusual for women to have very different perceptions of the same symptoms. Just as one person's

TABLE 2
CONDITIONS THAT MIMIC PMS

Fibrocystic breast changes
Endometriosis (pain and cramping)
Pelvic inflammatory disease
Dysmenorrhea (cramps secondary to other factors)
Thyroid disorders (too much or too little)
Endocrine disorders (abnormal adrenal function, etc.)
Clinical depression
Menopause
Dysthymic mood disorder (psychiatric diagnosis)
Birth-control-pill side effects
Eating disorders

perception of pain may be more or less than that of another, so certain symptoms may be experienced as more severe than others. The same symptom may be experienced differently by different persons. There is no cookbook recipe. Diagnosis and treatment has to be assessed individually. Imagine attaching a number to the severity of mood swings a woman experiences. Of two women who both have severe mood swings (based on my objective testing), Mabel may *feel* that her mood swings are severe, and Carol may *feel* that her mood swings are mild. That doesn't imply that Mabel is overly-sensitive to her moods and Carol is a Rock of Gibraltar. It is this all-important perception of severity that guides treatment. Mabel would be much more aggressive about seeking treatment than Carol, and rightly so.

Don't fall into the trap of thinking, "Well, Cousin Sally Mae has terrible PMS and she chants and takes gopher hair capsules and does great! Maybe I should get some of those gopher hair capsules!" It very rarely works that way. These changes are as unique to you as your own body. And so is the therapy. Your PMS has its own personality, but it is one that can be tamed. Don't forget you are "fearfully and wonderfully made," and God doesn't make junk.

Table 3 contains a partial list of common PMS symptoms. The scientific literature states that over 150 different symptoms have been associated with PMS. This is just a partial list, but it contains the most common complaints. Most women will only experience a few of these symptoms and, luckily, only to a mild degree.

The Brain Connection

I am frequently asked what causes PMS. The simple answer is, I don't know. In fact, the scientific community is unsure, but there are some theories. Research has established that there is an intimate link between estrogen and mental functioning. Estrogen has been shown to be mood-enhancing. It has many receptors in the brain and is also known to affect cognition and memory. The link appears to be a substance called serotonin. Serotonin is a brain hormone that is a regulator of many moods and emotions. It is a by-product of

Table 3
Symptoms of PMS

Physical	Emotional
Swelling and tenderness of the breasts	Increased appetite
Bloated feeling and temporary water weight gain	Food cravings
Skin breakouts or acne	Irritability
Swelling of hands and/or feet	Mood swings
Headaches	Insomnia
Nausea	Fatigue
Constipation	Forgetfulness or confusion
Diarrhea	Anxeity
Menstrual cramps	Sadness
Alcohol intolerance	Crying spells
Dizziness	Increased or decreased libido
Urinary urgency	Panic attacks
Backache	Increased aggresiveness
Vaginal irritation	Restlessness
Rashes	Social avoidance
Muscle aches	Anger
Leg cramps	Paranoia
Cold sweats	Difficulty concentrating
Hot flashes	Poor judgement
Sensitivity to light	Loneliness
Bruising	Indecision

L-tryptophan, an essential amino acid, and regulates such functions as sleep, menstrual cycles, and appetite.

Estrogen alters the metabolism or breakdown of serotonin that, in turn, is reflected in changes in emotions. Too little serotonin leads to symptoms of depression. That is why in many instances where there are hormonal shifts, such as puberty, postpartum, and menopause, there may be an associated effect on mood and behavior. More importantly, the estrogen/progesterone ratio can lead to an imbalance of these neurohormones. The connection is not completely clear, yet a great deal of research is being focused on this subject.

Another theory links PMS to a deficiency in a substance called beta-endorphin. This substance is chemically related to opium; however, beta-endorphin is produced naturally in your body. It can produce the "high" that some feel when exercising or can just be there to make you feel good. About a week before your period, beta-endorphin levels naturally decrease. As these levels decrease some researchers believe that the body undergoes a "mini opium withdrawal." Dr. Joseph Mortola, a psychiatrist at Beth Israel Hospital in Boston, states, "The withdrawal symptoms from opium and PMS symptoms are very similar–irritability, anger, and depression." This may explain why exercise is such an excellent remedy for many PMS problems.

This serotonin and endorphin connection doesn't explain all of the symptoms of PMS, however. Several other causative factors postulated are estrogen excess, progesterone deficiency, elevated prolactin (a hormone produced by the pituitary gland) levels, hypothyroidism, stress, depression, and nutritional factors. The most likely scenario is one in which a variety of factors are causative and interrelate to produce the symptom profile that is unique to that individual. The term *multifactorial* (see, I can use big words) best describes the etiology. There are most likely many different causes, all combining to give the unique PMS experience that you may experience. This is also why finding a specific treatment can be so frustrating.

Some fascinating work is being done on estrogen receptors in the brain. For a hormone to affect a cell it has to attach to that cell. This is the way it influences whether that cell produces a certain substance or acts in any other way. The way that the hormone attaches is by fitting into a space on the covering of the cell much like a puzzle piece fits into a puzzle. The space is called the receptor and it is specific for a certain puzzle piece. Once the puzzle piece fits into its place, the cell then performs a function that is specified by the completed puzzle. After a predetermined time the piece lifts out and travels back into the bloodstream, and that particular cell stops doing that particular task. Simple, right? It is actually very complex, and every time I learn more about how this system works I marvel at the awesome design of God.

The bottom line is that there are hormone receptors in the brain, and science is finding more and more about how estrogen, progesterone, and testosterone attach to them and affect moods, emotions, and feelings. For many this is not terribly important; however, it does validate scientifically what we have known anecdotally for many years. There is a definite relationship between hormones and behavior. It also tells us why many of the herbal and dietary approaches to controlling PMS work. They utilize this system to exert their effects. Many of the foodstuffs and herbs (particularly the phytoestrogens) fool the receptors into thinking they are estrogen and cause the cells to perform certain estrogen-like tasks. More about that later.

Making the Diagnosis

How do you know you have PMS? That may seem like a dumb question, yet one of the biggest problems in treating PMS is an inappropriate diagnosis by you or your health care provider. It only makes sense that to successfully treat a problem, you have to accurately identify the problem. It wouldn't make sense to treat Strep throat by putting a cast on the arm, and so it wouldn't make sense to treat PMS if you have another problem.

It is important to go back to the definition and review the critical components. Remember, PMS is a *predictable*, *recurrent* group of *bothersome* symptoms that occur in the second half of the menstrual cycle.

One of the best and most useful methods of diagnosing PMS is a symptom diary. Examples of symptom diaries abound. There are a variety of different forms available, but the basic idea is the same. Keeping an accurate day-by-day account of your feelings and symptoms is the fulcrum on which a correct diagnosis is balanced. There is no shortcut. The secret is the timing and repetitiveness of the problems, and the only way to demonstrate this is by consciously listening to your body and paying attention to the signs and symptoms you are experiencing. It really doesn't take much time, especially if it is a check-off form, but its usefulness is invaluable.

The symptom diary is important because it forces you to pay attention to your symptoms on a daily basis. It is a structured way to listen to your body. I have had many patients say that just *focusing on their feelings*, whether they are physical or emotional, can reduce the impact of symptoms. This is surprisingly difficult for many people to accomplish; however, the benefits are substantial. My experience indicates and most of the medical studies agree, that keeping a log for a minimum of three months is important. This allows for individual month-to-month variation and eliminates the isolated symptom that may occur in only one month. Remember, symptoms of PMS are predictable in onset and are repetitive.

The symptom diary also helps to pinpoint the timing of the problems in the cycle. The luteal phase of the cycle (the second half or days 14–28) is when classic PMS occurs. As I stated before, most women will describe a resolution of symptoms when the period starts. It is as though they are living in a dark cave during the height of their PMS and when their period begins the sun shines through a hole in the roof. I like this image because it reinforces the idea that these are recurring events that may create a darkness in mood, but the light is always there waiting to burst in.

The goal is to keep the room bathed in light. "Your eye is a lamp for your body. A pure eye lets sunshine into your soul. But an evil eye shuts out the light and plunges you into darkness. If the light you think you have is really darkness, how deep that darkness will be!" (Matt. 6:22–23) Jesus said to let our spiritual vision be made pure and God will send light in our darkened room. Our spiritual vision can be pure by focusing on God and His Word. "Your word is a lamp for my feet and a light for my path" (Ps. 119:105). It is important to focus on PMS symptoms to arrive at a diagnosis, but don't let it shift your vision from the bigger picture.

PMS is just one aspect of your life. Don't let it grow any more obtrusive than it already is by obsessing on its symptoms. "It is better to live alone in the corner of an attic than with a contentious wife in a lovely home" (Prov. 25:24).

One more note: Don't spend all of this time and effort and then forget to bring the diary to your health care worker! This is more important than any test he/she could do. I have had many women come to the office complaining of various problems that lead me to suspect PMS may be the source. Without the quantification and documentation of the symptoms, I often have to delay any treatment plan until I can verify my hunches. The symptom diary does this most effectively. Copy one or create your own in a calendar or journal and use it for three months. I can't emphasize enough that this is a vital piece of information, so it is worth your time and attention. Your doctor will praise you and your efforts. If he or she does not, find another doctor!

Beware

This brings me to a brief aside. There are many internists, family doctors, obstetricians, and gynecologists who do not like working with PMS. I know—I used to be one! The nature of the particular problem dictates the need for an inordinate amount of office time (or it should, to be properly dealt with). Many shy away from working with PMS because of the time involved in adequately treating it, or lack of knowledge regarding treatment options. For many busy doctors the PMS patient is a thorn in their side because there is no quick fix. The diagnosis and treatment cycle can easily stretch over several months and constitute many office visits.

It is important to find a doctor, nurse practitioner, counselor, or psychologist who has interest and experience in dealing with PMS. Where do you find such a person? Word of mouth. Talk to everyone and anyone who suffers from PMS, and they will be your best source of information. Then pray your insurance plan covers them and the problem! There are many wonderful health care providers who will take a special interest with you in making the diagnosis and then following through with a treatment plan. Do your homework, and you will be rewarded.

Seek Help

Once you are armed with the information regarding your symptoms, you are ready to go the next step. With the help of a competent, caring person, rule out the presence of other problems. One of the major reasons I included a chapter on PMS in this book is that many of the symptoms of PMS and the perimenopause are similar. It is easy for the layperson and the doctor to mistake one for the other. This is a major source of confusion to many who are in their mid- to late forties. Studies have shown that PMS may indeed worsen during this decade of life or even appear for the first time. What are these period irregularities? What are these mood swings? What are these hot flashes? PMS or menopause?

This is where some laboratory tests may be helpful. Let's take a minute and review the source of the changes for both of these transitions. In PMS there is a relative imbalance in estrogen and progesterone (in most cases), and the symptoms are largely due to estrogen dominance or estrogen's interaction with the hormone serotonin. (Remember, there are many other theorized etiologies, but for now let's focus on this known imbalance). Therefore, the goal is to restore this balance and alleviate the symptoms. Contrast that to menopause, where the symptoms are largely due to a decline in total estrogen and progesterone. In PMS there is still plenty of estrogen in your system, whereas in menopause there is a drop. It is not so much the absolute movement of estrogen up or down, but the ratio to other hormones and the secondary effects of estrogen that lead to symptoms. I hope it is obvious that the problems, while similar, may have different causes.

There are two hormones in particular that are helpful in making the distinction between PMS and menopause. They are FSH, follicle stimulating hormone, and LH, leutinizing hormone. These hormones are secreted by the pituitary gland and are intimately involved in the hormone balance that regulates normal ovulation. They have a unique inverse relationship with estrogen in that, when estrogen levels fall, the FSH and LH show a corresponding rise. Why not just measure the estrogen? Because the estrogen is secreted in a somewhat irregular fashion, a single value may not be accurate. A value drawn in the early morning may differ from a value done in the evening. The FSH and LH values are much steadier in their secretion; therefore, they provide a more meaningful set of numbers to analyze.

Simply stated, a high FSH and LH would indicate that a woman was either in or approaching menopause. There are certain times in the menstrual cycle when the LH may be high, so your doctor will need to know when in your cycle your blood is checked. Also, a single value may not give a clear picture, so occasionally the blood test will be repeated and the pattern will be analyzed. I won't bore you with a lot of statistics and numbers, because most numbers are meaningless unless taken in context with what is going on in the woman's body.

One of the first caveats we are taught in medical school is, "Don't treat a number, treat a *person*." That credo has kept me on track. That is not to say that these tests are not valuable. They are. But it is just as valuable to know what a person is feeling and experiencing. For example, Mrs. Brown may have a FSH of 40 MIU and Mrs. Black may have the exact same value, but their symptoms may be vastly different. This underscores a common theme throughout this book: Each person is unique, and you can't effectively work with someone without knowing her individual circumstances. The blood tests, placed in the context of the woman's history and symptoms, can greatly aid in making the distinction between PMS and perimenopause.

Action Challenge

Create your own symptom diary (a calendar will suffice) and commit to keeping an accurate account of your symptoms for three months.

CHAPTER FOUR

God's PMS-Relief Plan

Most people are not so concerned about the physiology of PMS as they are about symptom relief. They want to feel better, period! It is good and helpful to know the reason for a symptom, but it is even better to know what to do about it! The symptoms are what define PMS. It sounds simplistic, but without the symptoms there would be no PMS. I want to approach this in several ways. I will first talk in general about some things everyone can do to improve PMS, and then I will address specific solutions to individual symptoms. Remember that PMS is individualized; however, there are a few changes you can make that are universally helpful. The remainder of this chapter will be based on the assumption that you have correctly identified the problem as PMS. My prescription for success in PMS involves diet, lifestyle, potions, and prayer.

Diet

I hesitate to even use this word *diet* with all the baggage that it carries. Why would you do something that begins with the letters

D I E! Dieting is a way of making you miserable so you can live longer! It doesn't make sense. When I refer to dieting or diet here, I am talking generically about food intake. I use *diet* as a noun and not a verb. Included in this discussion will be foods, vitamins, and supplements. Again, remember that these are general recommendations, and it will be important to individualize their application to your situation and needs.

Foods were the original medications. Hippocrates, the father of modern medicine, said 2,500 years ago, "Let thy food be thy

FOOD PYRAMID

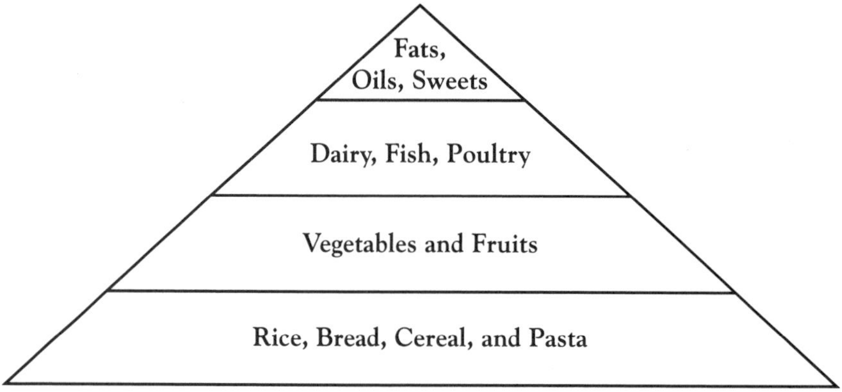

medicine." Before Prozac there were the hundreds of medicinal herbs and plants. The utilization of diet in the treatment of PMS (and all anxiety related disorders) is not new. The best "anti-PMS"diet plan can be described in one word, vegetarian. This is not a panacea, as there are many total vegetarians who have PMS. There are other important components to the dietary control of PMS, but the building blocks of successful treatment of PMS are fruits,vegetables, and fiber.

Studies have shown that a diet rich in fruits and vegetables and short on meat and dairy products promotes health and well-being. This is exceedingly applicable to PMS. I know you are probably saying, "I've heard all this before: Eat more veggies and fewer cows." Well, you have heard it often because, it's true. You only have to look to Genesis 1:29 to confirm this, God said, "See, I have given you every plant yielding seed that is upon the face of all the earth, and every tree with seed in its fruit; you shall have them for food." God was very clear in what constituted a healthy diet. Science has only now confirmed what the Bible has taught for hundreds of years.

Clinical Studies

In 1983, Dr. Guy Abraham published a study in the *Journal of Reproductive Medicine* in which he concluded that, compared to symptom-free women, PMS sufferers eat 62 percent more refined carbohydrates, 275 percent more refined sugar, 79 percent more dairy products, 78 percent more sodium, 53 percent less iron, 77 percent less manganese, and 52 percent less zinc.[1] Vegetarian diets have been shown to decrease the serum-free estrogen levels, mostly as a result of lower fat and higher fiber. Dr. Ronald Norris, in his book PMS, reports a key component of his dietary formula is to "sharply increase the intake of green leafy vegetables, whole grains, cereals, and legumes.[2]

Shifting your diet from one based on the old four food groups to one favoring the food pyramid is a more practical approach. Dramatic change in diet is difficult and somewhat unrealistic for many people, but a steady shift approximating a vegetarian diet will not only help improve PMS symptoms but will also alleviate many menopausal complaints. The long-term benefits are substantial.

Many resources are available that detail specific foods and recipes that constitute a vegetarian-based diet. One of the most effective and practical guides is Michael Murray's book *Encyclopedia of Natural Medicine*.[3] He talks about a Healthy Exchange System loosely based on the American Dietetic Association's Exchange System. It focuses on healthy, unprocessed, whole foods. The backbones of the system are vegetables, fruits, breads, cereals, legumes, and fats. A category for milk products and meats and fish is optional. The recommended dietary percentages are as follows:

Carbohydrates	60–70 percent of total calories
Fats	15–25 percent of total calories
Protein	15–20 percent of total calories
Dietary fiber	at least 50 g a day

These are simple recommendations, and this approach can be tailored to individual tastes and needs. Try one of the many excellent vegetarian cookbooks. Experiment and have fun! The goal is to make a permanent change in your dietary habits, not just a quick fix. The effect of a vegetarian diet will be not only a reduction or elimination of PMS symptoms but also a general feeling of increased vitality and well-being. In his book *What the Bible Says about Healthy Living*, Dr. Rex Russell says, "God has been concerned about our health since creation, not just since Moses gave the law. Because he created us, it makes sense that He should know best what makes us healthy."[4]

Fat Is Not Where It's At

Vegetarian-based diets form the foundation of a successful dietary approach to PMS; however, it doesn't stop there. It is almost as important to learn what not to put in your mouth as it is to know what to eat.

Reduce your fat intake, in particular saturated fats. Fats are separated into saturated and unsaturated depending on differences in their chemical structure. The practical distinction is that saturated fat consumption has been linked to the development of heart disease, while unsaturated fat is less likely to cause a problem. You have to have some fat in your diet. There are many essential body functions that require different fats. The problem arises when we overdo it. (Remember the idea of balance.)

The most effective way to decrease the saturated fat content in your diet is to eliminate as much meat as possible since it is a major source of saturated fat. A study by D. Y. Jones in 1987 showed a marked improvement of PMS symptoms in women with a low fat diet.[5] Other studies have shown a decrease in serum estrogen levels in women who consumed 25 percent of calories from fat as opposed to women who ate 40 percent calories from fats.[6]

Nuts and seeds do contain a high percentage of fat; however, the fat calories are largely derived from polyunsaturated essential fatty acids. These fats are not only less harmful, but as the name implies, they are essential for proper body functioning. Dr. Ronald Norris, noted PMS researcher, states that polyunsaturated fats should constitute less than 20 percent of your total daily intake.[7] The public is besieged with conflicting information about fat consumption. There is no question that a low-fat diet helps in PMS and contributes to your overall health. Udo Erasmus, Ph.D, in his book *Fats that Kill, Fats that Heal*, states,

> The fact is that some fats are absolutely required for health, while others are detrimental. Some fats heal, and others kill. Whether fat heals or kills depends on several factors. What kind of fat is it? How has it been treated—is it fresh, has it been exposed to light, oxygen, heat, hydrogen, water, acid, base, or metals like copper and iron? How old is it? How much was eaten? What balance of different fats do we get? If we get the right kinds of fats in the right amounts and balances, and prepare them using the right methods, they build our health and keep us healthy. The wrong kinds of fats, the wrong amounts or balances, or even the right kinds of fats wrongly prepared cause degenerative diseases that we call fatty degeneration. Other nutrients can also cause fatty degeneration, and so can lack of certain essential nutrients. We can reverse diseases of fatty degeneration by making appropriate changes in fat choices, preparation, and consumption and by supporting these important changes with attention to other nutrients in our food supply.[8]

Sweet Revenge

Mom always said, "Watch your sweets." And mom was right! Sugar intake has been associated with higher estrogen levels. Women with elevated sugar consumption have been shown to have markedly more intense PMS symptoms. It is interesting that a lot of problems associated with hypoglycemia (low blood sugar) mimic PMS symptoms. Research indicates that, especially during the luteal phase of the menstrual cycle, the body's reaction to drops in blood sugar levels is magnified. Normally after a meal the blood sugar rises as carbohydrates from the meal are broken down and make their way into the bloodstream. This triggers the release of insulin, a hormone responsible for taking the blood glucose and transferring it into cells and tissues for storage or use.

In some women during the luteal phase of their cycle this insulin response is magnified, and the blood sugar levels are driven too low. This results in symptoms of low blood sugar such as anxiety, sweating, fatigue, and palpitations. The key is to limit sugar intake in the diet to minimize the insulin overreaction. Trying to avoid these peaks and valleys in sugar levels is helpful in controlling PMS. How do you do this? By eating frequent small meals throughout the day and avoiding high sugar foods.

The interaction between the menstrual cycle and insulin secretion is an example of how all the body systems work together. You can't just eliminate your body's other functions while you isolate the PMS changes; they are all intertwined. A helpful approach is to eat smaller, frequent meals (to avoid sudden sugar loads) and to stay away from high sugar foods. (And we all know what those are, don't we?)

What is the "best" sweetener? The Bible is clear. Honey. It is mentioned over fifty times in most translations, and most are of the nature of Proverbs 24:13: "My child, eat honey, for it is good, and the honeycomb is sweet to the taste." The reference is to unprocessed honey. Does this mean you can sit at home during a PMS craving and eat a jar of honey and not suffer any ill effects? Heed the warning of Proverbs 25:27: "Just as it is not good to eat too much honey, it is not good for people to think about all the honors they deserve." Dr. Rex Russell summarizes the practical consumption of sugar:

> Enjoy honey, fruit juices, barley sweetener and black strap molasses. One tablespoon of honey is equivalent in sweetness to five tablespoons of sugar. When cooking with honey, reduce the total amount of other liquids by one-quarter cup per cup of honey. Also, lower the baking temperature 50 degrees to prevent over baking. Enjoy the things created for food that contain natural sugars. Enjoy complex carbohydrates. If you must eat sugar, make sure you eat plenty of fiber and nutrients along with it.[9]

Other substances to avoid are caffeine, salt, and alcohol. All of these "foods" have been associated with an intensification of PMS symptoms. Caffeine especially can increase breast tenderness and, surprisingly, fatigue! High salt intake is notorious for promoting fluid retention and bloating. Limit yourself; take away your salt shaker (we don't even own one) and get into the habit of reading labels. With the new laws it is much easier to discover the sodium content of prepackaged, processed foods.

I will spend more time in Section 3 dealing specifically with foods and how they relate to midlife and menopause.

In summary, here is a proper diet for effective control of PMS: If it tastes good spit it out. The primary foodstuff for daily consumption is cardboard! If this doesn't work for you, then a reasonable foundation of a vegetarian-based diet, elimination of caffeine, salt, and most sweets, will start you on the right path.

Vitamins

Vitamins are an essential component of any healthy nutritional program. Many important vitamins are obtained through eating the right foods, but often supplements are needed. I am an advocate of using multivitamins and minerals to supplement our often-inadequate diet. Most multivitamins contain a reasonable dosage of common ingredients (based on the percentage of average daily requirements as established by the government). The two vitamins I will discuss in the context of PMS often need to be used in addition to a multivitamin because the required effective dose is higher than found in most single multivitamin combinations.

Vitamin B6 (pyridoxine) is one of the B vitamins. A study by Barr in 1984 showed an improvement in 84 percent of patients with PMS when treated with B6 as compared to a placebo. This was a double-blind study, which is the gold standard in research.[10] An excellent review of vitamin B6 therapy was published in the *British Journal of Obstetrics and Gynecology* in 1990, which showed that a majority of studies evaluating vitamin B6 therapy in PMS were positive.[11] Some of the studies reviewed showed no positive effect, however, so it is clear that this approach does not work for all women.

It is important to remember this caveat in dealing with any vitamin or herbal approach: The treatments don't work overnight! The key is persistence. If they are right for you, you will only begin to notice their effect after one to two months of continual use. This means using them consistently and in the proper dosages for an adequate amount of time is paramount in assessing their effectiveness.

What doses of vitamin B6 are appropriate? Based on clinical studies, using 50 to 100 mg a day achieves the therapeutic results in those with whom it will help. This is a vitamin that has to be used wisely because excessive doses (1,500-2,000 mg) have been associated with nerve toxicity. My own routine involves starting with 50 mg a day, and using that for at least a month before considering any increase. Vitamin B6 is found in nature in yeast extract (herbaforce), sesame seeds, sesame seed oil, carrots, celery, barley, okra, almonds, turnip greens, olives, bananas, onions, leeks, turnips, grapes, and honey.

Vitamin E is the second supplement that has been shown in multiple studies to reduce some of the symptoms of PMS. In particular, vitamin E improves some of the physical complaints such as breast tenderness and fatigue. Several double-blind studies in 1983 and 1984 showed improvement in these symptoms, anxiety, and depression.[12] Note that in these studies vitamin E use was compared to a placebo. Why is this important? Research has shown a rather marked response to placebo in treating PMS, so for a comparison to be valid you must have this control group. Otherwise it is impossible to say whether the effect was due to the tested substance or the power of suggestion.

I especially like vitamin E for the relief of breast tenderness. I have found that it sometimes takes up to 800 units a day to get satisfactory reduction in breast tenderness, and it tends to work best if taken on a daily basis. It is best to use the *d-alpha* tocopherol (the fancy chemical name for vitamin E) as opposed to the *dl-alpha* tocopherol, as the former is the natural occurring vitamin and the latter is a synthetic, less-effective compound. Vitamin E can be found in nature in fish, egg yolk, cereal, fruit oils, cotton seed, corn, peanuts, and watercress. Abundant sources of vitamin E are spinach, lettuce, alfalfa, and most leafy salad greens. In addition vitamin E helps prevent blood clots and has been associated with a reduction of heart disease.

Supplements

Included in this category of supplements are minerals and trace elements that either directly or indirectly play a role in PMS. They are important in its alleviation because of their interaction with the body systems that control PMS symptoms. The first of these substances is calcium. Calcium is especially important in the perimenopausal years as its intake during this time may affect os-teoporosis risks. What is done during this time may dramatically affect later years. Adequate calcium intake even as early as the teen years has been shown to affect total bone mass entering menopause.

Some studies have suggested that calcium supplements in the range of 1,000 mg a day may improve PMS symptoms.[13] One review in 1983 suggested that extra calcium might actually increase some symptoms. Most recently, in 1997, a large randomized study again confirmed that there was an improvement in overall PMS symptoms in calcium users as opposed to nonusers.[14]

A large, randomized, double-blind study (the gold standard in research) published in 1998 looked at 497 premenopausal women with PMS. This study used 1,200 mg of calcium carbonate (Turns, Os-cal, Caltrate, etc.) daily over three cycles. By the third cycle about 48 percent of calcium users showed a reduction in symptoms. Twenty-nine percent of women given calcium had a greater than 75 percent improvement in their symptoms as compared to 16 percent who were given the placebo. It is interesting that 36 percent of the people given the placebo (sugar pill) showed a 50 percent improvement in symptoms.[15] This illustrates the power of the mind in controlling many PMS problems. Never underestimate the power of the placebo!

My own bias is that most women need to be thinking about extra calcium intake at this stage of their life (either through diet or supplements) anyway, so it makes healthy sense to incorporate this into your overall wellness approach, PMS or not. There is more about calcium in the chapter on osteoporosis.

Magnesium

An article in a European medical journal in 1994 suggested that magnesium plays a major role in PMS.[16] This illustrates the multifactorial nature of the etiology of this syndrome. There is no single cause of PMS, but several factors combine to produce the spectrum of maladies. The goal of you and your health care worker is to find what major influences exist in your body.

An article in a major obstetrics and gynecology journal in 1991 found that magnesium supplementation was an effective treatment for PMS.[17] Magnesium appears to work alone; however, other studies show that it may be more effective when combined with other vitamins and nutrients. The range of magnesium supplementation that has been effective in various studies varies from 300–500 mg a day. (This nonspecific range illustrates the problem with many studies on vitamins and nutrients). Good natural sources of magnesium include apples, beet greens, blackberries, blueberries, celery, cherries, cabbage, coconuts, figs, grapes, lemons, limes, oats, oranges, peas, plums, potatoes, prunes, squash, and turnips. One possible bothersome side effect from high dose supplement preparations is a potential laxative effect.

Zinc

Another important mineral in the treatment of PMS is zinc. Zinc acts as a cofactor for many hormones, and its presence in adequate amounts is essential for the proper functioning of these substances.

Most healthy diets will provide plenty of zinc. Some special restricted diets may benefit from a zinc supplement, and adequate zinc is contained in most multivitamins. Studies in 1987 and 1991 confirm that a multivitamin and mineral supplement can produce a 70 percent reduction in PMS symptoms.[18] Nature's sources of zinc include celery, barley, okra, almonds, collards, olives, beet greens, yogurt, papaya, sesame seeds, cucumbers, kale, and apples.

The food we eat is the fuel that drives the system. No one would debate the absolutely wonderful results that are experienced when you work in concert with your innate, God-given healing potential. A good and proper diet does just that. Remember that the two greatest actions you can take to promote healing in any situation are to provide the body what it needs to function properly and eliminate those things that block this intrinsic ability.

Food and supplements are another steppingstone to utilize in crossing the treacherous PMS waters. Now, let's look at lifestyle changes that will both promote health and remove negative influences.

Lifestyle Changes

My dad told me years ago that anything worth having is worth working for. I didn't like hearing that, as I would often try to find the shortest path to an end. I found out quickly that the shortest and easiest route is often neither! This certainly applies to lifestyle changes that help with PMS.

Bill Norman writes in *Leadership* magazine about a business consultant who decided to landscape his grounds. He hired an extremely knowledgeable woman with a doctorate in horticulture. Because the business consultant was very busy and traveled a lot, he kept emphasizing to her the need to create his garden in a way that would require little or no maintenance on his part. He insisted on automatic sprinklers and other labor saving devices. Finally she stopped and said, "There's one thing you need to deal with before we go any further. If there's no gardener, there's no garden!"

Likewise, there are no labor saving devices for growing a garden of spiritual virtue. Becoming a person of spiritual fruitfulness requires time, attention, and care. In the same way, overcoming PMS or menopausal problems requires a long-term commitment. There is no successful and lasting quick fix.

You may already be exercising, avoiding caffeine and alcohol, getting counseling, using prayer, or developing stress management techniques. If so, great! Keep it up! If not, I want to explain how each one of these lifestyle changes can help in the midlife and beyond. I will expand on many of these ideas and activities later since they also apply to menopause, yet I want to spend some time introducing the topics now because of their application to PMS.

Exercise

If you could take a pill that made you look better, feel better, act better, lose weight, reduce your chance of heart disease, breast cancer and stroke, reduce or eliminate PMS and menopausal problems, and do all of this without any side effects, would you take it? Of course you would. Well, that pill exists. It's called exercise, and it takes about 45 minutes to swallow!

I am convinced that exercise is the fountain of youth. I devote an entire chapter to the how-to and the why later on, but for now, let's look at the reasons why exercise helps in PMS.

Virtually every study that has looked at exercise during the luteal phase of the cycle has shown a significant improvement in PMS symptoms. Several recent studies compared women who exercised on a regular basis with those who were sedentary (that word even sounds ominous) and found that the exercisers had much better scores for concentration, moods, and physical symptoms like cramping and pain.[19] Most suspect that this response is mediated through two mechanisms.

First, exercise is a well-known stress reducer. It is known that stress can act as a modifier of PMS feelings. The more stress you are under the more intense the PMS symptoms can be, and the converse is also true. The less stress you have, the lower the intensity of PMS. Covert Bailey writes in *Smart Exercise*, "If your kids are screaming, the soup is burning on the stove, and the cat is sampling your bridge party *hors d'oeuvres*, you'll handle it better if you have been exercising regularly." He goes on to say, "What is stressful to a sedentary person is less stressful to an exercised person."[20]

Second, exercise has been shown to increase the bloodstream circulation of chemicals called endorphins. These substances are responsible for blunting pain perception and causing improved moods. Many distance runners talk about the "runner's high" they achieve. This is an endorphin-mediated response. The increased level of endorphins in the body secondary to exercise can blunt many of the pain and mood changes of PMS.

The greatest benefit in reducing PMS problems is achieved by those women who exercise throughout the cycle. Studies have even shown some improvements may occur with exercise only during the second half of the cycle. Yes, there is even hope for you chronic couch potatoes. Covert Bailey again summarizes the benefits of exercise on stress by saying, "Aerobic exercise is a stress that make us tough enough to handle all other stresses."[21]

How much exercise is enough? Most studies show a benefit for PMS with activity of three days a week for 45 minutes at a time. This applies mainly to aerobic exercise where you are doing something that elevates your heart rate to a target point and maintains it there for the duration of the exercise.

There are many ways to calculate your maximum heart rate; with the simplest being 220 minus your age. This gives a basic ballpark value for the maximum heart rate. Most aerobic exercise is achieved by keeping your level of exercise strenuous enough to keep your pulse at 60-80 percent of your calculated maximum heart rate. The range of 60-80 percent is called the target heart rate. If you don't want to stop and count your pulse, there are many heart rate monitors available that you can wear during exercise that will do this for you.

This may sound complicated, but most people (especially new exercisers) can easily achieve this level of exertion by a brisk walk, (not a casual stroll in the park) any type of good aerobic class or tape, running, or biking. Make it fun, make it convenient, but make it mandatory. Get your spouse or a friend to do it with you. Chances are they need it as much or more than you do! The Delaney sisters wrote in the *Christian Reader*, "God only gave you one body, so you better be nice to it. Exercise, because if you don't, by the time you're our age [103 and 105], you'll be pushing up daisies."[22]

Eliminating harmful behaviors that interfere with the body's ability to function properly is a common theme throughout this book. Accentuate the positive, and eliminate the negative! (Makes me want to break into song.) Three culprits are especially prevalent and harmful in dealing with PMS, and should be minimized or eliminated.

Java Junkies

Caffeine is the most common legal addictive drug in use today. Table 4 lists the caffeine content of several common drinks and foods.

It is surprising how much caffeine invades our daily routine. It can worsen the symptoms of PMS, including breast tenderness, heart

TABLE 4*
CAFFEINE CONTENT

Source		Milligrams of Caffeine
Coffee	Drip, 8 oz	150-180
	Perked, 8 oz	125
	Instant, 8 oz	30-120
	Decaffeinated, 8 oz	2-8
Tea	Brewed, 8 oz	20-100
	Instant, 8 oz	30-70
Soft drinks	Mountain Dew	54
	Colas	366
Other	**Hot cocoa, 8 oz**	**4-8**
	Chocolate, 1 oz	14
	Vivarin, 1 tablet	200
	No-Doz, 1 tablet	100
	Excedrin, 1 tablet	75
	Anacin, 1 tablet	32
	Midol, 1 tablet	32

*Source: Data from C. Bailey, *Smart Exercise*, (New York: Houghton Mifflin, 1994), 209.

palpitations, fatigue, bladder problems, and hot flashes. But what would we do without those Maxwell House moments? Chances are, a lot better! Some women are so sensitive to the effects of caffeine that one soda or one cup of coffee can elicit a multitude of symptoms. I caution you that stopping cold turkey will lead to some temporary ill effects such as headaches and moodiness, yet the eventual payoff will greatly offset these short-lived inconveniences. Make a plan to taper the withdrawal. Tell someone of your intentions and have them hold you accountable. Make a plan and stick to it. With a little effort, you can stop being that java junkie.

Alcohol

Alcohol has an interesting association with PMS. There are a lot of anecdotal reports of women self-medicating with alcohol during their PMS periods. It is their attempt to lessen the symptoms; however, most would report that over time they actually noticed an intensification of symptoms with alcohol use.

One woman I interviewed gave an interesting account of her road to alcohol abuse. She rationalized her drinking, beginning at age fourteen, as a reaction to her mother's PMS symptoms! She related that during "that time" her mother would become hostile, abusive, and uncaring. The daughter's drinking was a survival mechanism to combat the horrible circumstances at home. She soon realized that this was just adding to the overall problem and was doing nothing to alleviate the situation. She also began to see certain PMS behaviors in herself, so a part of her recovery was to treat not only the alcohol abuse but also the PMS symptoms.

This reinforces the idea that none of these symptoms exists in isolation. In dealing with PMS, or any other health matter, a person's entire situation has to be evaluated. The bottom line is that for most women alcohol use during the PMS cycle will only make symptoms worse. Samuel Johnson wrote, "One of the disadvantages of wine is that it makes a man mistake words for thoughts." Proverbs 20:1 states, "Wine produces mockers; liquor leads to brawls. Whoever is led astray by drink cannot be wise."

Stress Me Out

Stress plays a momentous role in PMS and midlife in general. It is the volume control on the symptom stereo. In times of increased stress a woman, who may otherwise not experience PMS, may see those problems appear. Likewise, those who routinely suffer from PMS can see their suffering greatly magnified in stressful situations. "A nagging wife is as annoying as the constant dripping on a rainy day. Trying to stop her complaints is like trying to stop the wind or hold something with greased hands." (Prov. 27:15)

Stress is pervasive throughout society. If you had to use one word to characterize life in the twentieth century, it is stress. Some researchers have suggested that up to 70 percent of visits to the doctor are directly or indirectly due to stress and anxiety. I get stressed just thinking and writing about all the stress! For years I was nonchalant in dealing with patients and stress, and I had a "just deal with it" attitude. However, it has become clear that to follow a mission of facilitating healing I can't ignore this ever-present, serious threat to health.

Hans Selye, noted psychologist and pioneer in the field of stress research, defined stress as the nonspecific response of the organism to any pressure or demand. The operative phrase in this definition is "nonspecific response." It is the perception of the person that defines a stress or stressor. Dr. Martin Seligman, who has done extensive research on optimism and health, writes that it is not the potential stressor itself but how it is perceived that is important. He goes on to say that how you handle the pressure or demand will determine whether or not it will lead to stress. I don't need to rehash all of the medical problems associated with stress. Most of them are well known.

The million-dollar question is, how do you reduce stress in your life? What can you do, beginning today, that can have an impact on lowering your stress level? Notice I didn't say how could you eliminate stress, for I don't believe you can totally eliminate it. In fact, I am convinced that stress can be beneficial. After all, a diamond is only coal under stress.

Deal with It

How do you view stress with a positive perspective and use it to enhance body function instead of thwarting it? The most effective guidance for stress management lies in the Word. First, honestly and realistically identify the stressor. Look at John 8:32: "And you will know the truth, and the truth will set you free."

This may sound simple but may be the most difficult aspect of dealing with stress. In this instance the truth is the source of the stress. Is it internal? Is it external? Is it physical? Is it psychological? For example, for many, a job promotion is a happy event. However, if there are perceived conflicts with increased job expectations or demands, the "good stress" resulting from the promotion can be negated. Even though the money and status is better, the stress is magnified. The problem or source of stress may not be the actual job, but more the fear of failure. Often the source of the problem is so buried that to uncover it is a frightening task. The act of introspection may create a great deal of perceived stress in and of itself.

Introspection is an absolutely vital step, however, because the road to effective management of the stress is only successfully traveled by correctly identifying its source. That way you don't fall into the trap of simply treating symptoms and not causes. Treating symptoms is like a dog chasing his tail: You usually get nowhere and end up mad! Inevitably, it is only a temporary fix and can often even contribute to the problem. I won't downplay the difficulty in doing this, and often you must seek the assistance of others.

Either a well-trained Christian counselor or a pastor can be an invaluable resource. A good counselor can act as a mirror and reflect your fears and anxieties and put them into context. Don't be afraid to call on these people. Seeking the truth, as John points out, is the first step in setting you free from the bondage of stress. Take inventory of the major stressors in your life. Again many of us are not able to do this successfully by ourselves. Pray, listen, and act. Ask God to provide you with assistance. In prayer you are not reminding God that you need help in identifying your sources of stress. (He is already aware of this.) You are reminding yourself that you need God's help in life.

So the first and most important step in dealing with stress is to seek out and identify the source of the stress. Stress may come from external sources or, more likely, from within. Stress is simply an emotional and/or physical response to some type of stimulus. Charles Swindoll said, "Life is 10 percent what happens to us and 90 percent how we deal with it." Stress is a reaction to internal or external stimulus. Stress is an intangible emotion that is defined by the one experiencing the stimuli.

How you see things and how you react to them makes all the difference in terms of how much stress you experience. You control the physiological and psychological responses to events; therefore, you control what is "stressful." In other words, if you are having an argument with your spouse about money, how you process the words, how you react to the expressions, and how you think about the consequences determines the stress level you feel. There is no tangible item that is "stress." You can't hold it or touch it. It is a way of thinking that is manifested by emotional and physical symptoms. You perceive a situation as stressful if it elicits certain feelings and emotions.

The point is that you do have control over your perceptions. You have control over your thoughts. You choose to perceive something as stressful or nonstressful. You can use those thoughts to your advantage. This gives great hope to a Christian who has many sources to help influence her thoughts.

An example of the positive channeling of stress is the athlete who thrives on competition. No one would argue that a fiercely fought athletic struggle is stressful; however, many can use this stress to their advantage. They acknowledge that the situation is tough, but they have confidence in their ability and, more importantly, they know they can control their thoughts and behavior. They can take this stressful situation and turn it into a victory.

You can do the same thing in your daily life. You can decide if you are going to let a stressor control your thoughts or if you are going to use that energy to be a winner. Where do you get the ability to control your thoughts, feelings, and emotions? And how do you do it? Look at Paul's letter to the Philippians: "Fix your thoughts on what is true and honorable and right. Think about things that are pure and lovely and admirable. Think about things that are excellent and worthy of praise." (Phil. 4:8)

From where does the power come? Directly from God. God knows our thoughts and wants us to be clear in our thinking. God also has the power to help us in choosing to control our perceptions. Isaiah 55:8 illustrates this power: "'My thoughts are completely different from yours,' says the LORD. 'And my ways are far beyond anything you could imagine. For just as the heavens are higher than the earth, so are my ways higher than your ways and my thoughts higher than your thoughts.'" He is the ultimate power; however, His strength is available to us through His grace. How do we know this? Paul writes in the letter to the Colossians, "Let heaven fill your thoughts. Do not think only about things down here on earth." (Colossians 3:2)

It seems obvious that Paul's instruction could not be carried out if God were not willing to give us the strength and guidance to do so. We access this strength through prayer and through interaction with those trained in providing guidance. Here is where a community of believers can play a major role. I do not share the First Lady's admonition that it takes a village to raise a child, but I do believe that an effective deterrent to stress in your life is a supportive network of friends or family.

Daily in my office I see people who are struggling with all manner of stressors and toils. Life is tough. Yet, inevitably, two characteristics of the survivors stand out. First, they have a strong spiritual faith. Whether Christian, Moslem, Jewish, Hindu, or any other person of faith, they have a firm moral and ethical foundation upon which to make decisions and deal with adversity. Second, they have supportive family and friends who provide comfort and advice. There is no substitute for someone being there to listen, hold, cry, or celebrate. "A friend is always loyal, and a brother is born to help in time of need" (Prov. 17:17). "If one person falls, the other can reach out and help. But people who are alone when they fall are in real trouble. And on a cold night, two under the same blanket can gain warmth from each other. But how can one be warm alone? A person standing alone can be attacked and defeated, but two can stand back-to-back and conquer. Three are even better, for a triple-braided cord is not easily broken." (Eccl. 4:10–12)

Summary

Effective stress management is a two-fold process. First, identify the stressor and its source. Second, confront it. This is a healthy approach and certainly one that will endure beyond the short term. There are certain situations in which some medications are justified, but only on a short-term basis and only to get you to a point mentally that you can begin the real work of stress relief. Anti-anxiety medications can be helpful, but always remember they are treating a symptom and not a cause. They are like a psychic Band-Aid, not a permanent solution.

Whole books have been written about the complex topic of stress management; however, I hope I have been able to introduce some basic concepts and allow you to develop this as it applies to your life. Jon Kabat-Zinn, in his book *Full Catastrophe Living*, says, "It can be particularly helpful to keep in mind from moment to moment that it is not so much the stressors in our lives but how we see them and what we do with them that determines how much we are at their mercy. If we can change the way we see, we can change the way we respond."[23] The key to handling stress lies in understanding your dependence on God and submitting to His guidance. God has given us the ability to make choices about our thoughts and feelings. Choose wisely! A reduction in stress leads directly to a diminution in PMS problems.

The Psalmist writes, "My flesh and my heart may fail, but God is the strength of my heart and my portion forever." First Peter 5:6–7 states the case succinctly and simply: "Humble yourselves therefore under the mighty hand of God, so that He may exalt you in due time. *Cast all your anxiety on Him, because He cares for you*" (emphasis mine).

Potions

For every person who has bad PMS, there is a homegrown "potion" that they have tried. It is inevitable that in a situation where there is no one single identifiable cause there naturally will follow a variety of solutions. This is evident in PMS therapies. Vitamin and dietary regimens may not work for some. Everyone will not respond to herbal, hormonal, or psychoactive drug combinations. The process is often trial and error. In many cases a combination of diet, exercise stress management and " potions" works best. I define *potions* as any regimen involving herbs, plants, or natural medicines. I use this word tongue-in-cheek to illustrate the variety of options, not to imply any negative connotations.

Approach PMS treatment with an open mind—with the goal being a happy, healthy life. Don't limit your frame of reference. Open your mind and your heart to the possibilities. Dr. H. C. A. Vogel, noted naturopath and author of *The Nature Doctor*, writes, "Good health involves more than taking remedies. If we want to live healthy, happy, and joyful lives, we must endeavor to re-establish the proper relationship between ourselves-the whole body and mind-and nature. There is no other way to lead a happy and satisfied life. If we violate nature its harmony is destroyed, for we are a part of nature. In the same way, all medical research is a waste of time if these holistic interrelationships are not taken into consideration."[24] When I read this, I substitute "God" for "nature" and the meaning is clearer in the context of my own beliefs.

There are three factors in choosing potions that must always be kept in mind. First, they usually don't work overnight. Even prescription medicines often take several cycles to exert their influence. There is no quick fix that is safe and long term. It is not unusual for the herbal preparations to take from four to six weeks to exhibit their effectiveness. The biggest mistakes people make are not taking the herbs long enough or in the right doses.

Second, the regimens should be approached in a step fashion. Don't try every herbal regimen all at once. If you feel better, how will you know which is the effective herb? Is it an individual herb? Or is it a combination? Take it in a slow, logical progression so you can properly assess what is working for you.

And third, don't rely solely on these potions. Remember this is a combined approach involving your whole person. Don't leave out the exercise or stress management simply because you are taking some pill or using a cream. A common mistake is relying on only one component of the healing triad. Don't forget that health is a balance between mind, body, and spirit, and this especially applies to PMS. It is easy to get caught up in the latest fad treatment, whether it is an herb or diet or philosophy, and lose focus on the bigger picture.

Since my bias leans toward the "natural" approach, I will discuss these various options first. Herbal remedies are as old as humanity. Some of the earliest written records are from Egyptian medical "texts" that espouse the benefits of certain herbal preparations. In biblical times oils, balms, and herbs were as much a part of traditional medicine as antibiotics and x-rays are today. Herbs had an especially prominent place as dietary supplements as seen in the instructions for the Passover meal in Exodus 12:7: "That evening everyone must eat roast lamb with bitter herbs and bread made without yeast." In this particular context, the use of herbs is symbolic of the bitterness of the Jewish captivity and not for medicinal purposes, but it illustrates the prevalence and familiarity of the people with various herbs. They were commonplace.

Ezekiel 47:12 says, "All kinds of fruit trees will grow along both sides of the river. The leaves of these trees will never turn brown and fall, and there will always be fruit on their branches. There will be a new crop every month, without fail! For they are watered by the river flowing from the Temple. *The fruit will be for food and the leaves for healing*" (emphasis mine).

The use of herbs to treat certain medical problems has persisted through the ages. It is an accurate assumption that if there were not some validity to their effectiveness they would not be around now. In fact, herbs and plants were the predominant medicines until this century. We, in the United States, are in the midst of a revival in herbalism. The use of herbal medicines is quickly marching back into the mainstream. Evidence for this is the publication in 1998 of the first edition of the *PDR for Herbal Medicines*. For years the PDR has been the gold standard for doctors in prescribing medications and researching side effects and dosages. The introduction of this manual characterizes the resurgence of interest in herbs. "Almost overnight, herbal remedies have become a major factor in American health. Botanicals with names like Ginseng, St. John's Wort, and Ma Huang have suddenly become household words across the United States. Sales of herbal remedies are doubling every four years. And, as herbs move out of the health food stores and into mainstream supermarkets and drugstores, the trend toward self-medication with 'natural' supplements seems certain to accelerate."[25]

I am going to present *only* the herbal therapies that either my patients and I have had personal experience with or for which I have documented clinical research from America and Europe to support their effectiveness. One of the major drawbacks to the use of herbal medicines is the unsubstantiated claims by some of usage and efficacy.

This is not meant to be a comprehensive discourse on all available options. There are other approaches, many others. This will provide you with a springboard to launch your journey to healing. These options work. Have confidence that many women have used them, and if used properly, their safety is unmatched.

Licorice Root

The first of the herbal approaches is licorice root (Glycyrrhiza Glabra). This isn't the stuff you buy in the candy store! Its use in female disorders dates back to medieval times. Licorice has long been used for stomach and gastrointestinal problems. Hippocrates, the father of modern medicine, used this "sweet root" frequently, and Hildegard of Bingen, probably the best-known medieval herbalist, included it in her Materia Medica. I am not aware of any good double-blind studies that looked specifically at its use for PMS; however, I have seen it be successful in treating some of the associated symptoms.

In particular, licorice root is helpful in conditions secondary to fluid retention or edema, from ankle swelling to headaches to that puffy sensation that occurs around the period. A study published in the 1991 *New England Journal of Medicine* showed that licorice root acts to block the effect of aldosterone.[26] Aldosterone is a hormone produced by the adrenal glands that is responsible for regulating the amount of fluid in the tissues and bloodstream. This hormone is elevated in some sufferers of PMS, especially those with a lot of bloating and swelling. The licorice root acts to block the aldosterone receptors, thus balancing this overproduction. Because of this action, it should be used with caution in people with renal disease, heart disease, or high blood pressure. I have seen patients eliminate excess fluid and water-weight gain on a standardized regimen of 250 mg three times a day taken on the days of the luteal phase (days 14–28).

Black Cohosh

Black cohosh (Cimicifuga Racemosa) is another herb that has long been used for a variety of menstrual disorders. It was a major ingredient in the famous "vegetable compound" from Lydia Pinkham. Native American herbalists gave many of its uses to us. I will look at it in more depth when I talk about different approaches to menopause, since it has its most popular and proven effectiveness there. A German study in 1964 utilized a product that is a standard extract of black cohosh called Remifemin, and showed a reduction in feelings of depression and anxiety in women suffering from PMS. This brand name is now available in the United States and is in many drug and health food stores. I have seen moderate success with its use in women who tend to have a preponderance of emotional symptoms with PMS. It is generally dosed at one tablet twice a day during the luteal phase. It is felt, that because black cohosh is a phytoestrogen, it balances the estrogen/progesterone ratio and thus improves the emotional impact of the luteal phase shift.

Chasteberry

Probably the most tested and popular herbal approach to PMS is chasteberry extract (Vitex Agnus-Castus). It is one of the most widely-used products in Europe for PMS. Vitex has a fascinating history, from being used by temple priestesses in ancient Greece to suppress libido to being sold in Egyptian bazaars as a "calming agent in hysteria." Two German studies in the early 1990s looked at over 1,500 women with PMS and reported that over 90 percent showed some improvement in their symptoms with the use of chasteberry extract.[27] The dosage in these studies ranged from 175 mg to 225 mg (standardized extract) a day in capsule form, and this was taken daily-as opposed to the previously listed herbs that were used only in the luteal cycle.

Note this about quality and reliability: As this surge in interest in herbal products began, there was an associated rise in the number of companies producing their versions of products. Many poor quality producers jumped on the bandwagon. In fact, many of the poor reputations that some herbal products acquired were directly related to shoddy manufacturing, not the herb itself.

Herbs are not regulated by any agency-yet. The only quality control is what the individual company requires, and this is totally self-determined and self-contained. You have to do your homework. You have to look at the company's literature, ask questions, and choose a company that you feel comfortable with. In selecting and using vitamin or herbal products, pick a manufacturer with which you are pleased and try to get all your "potions" from them. Not only will this simplify your acquisitions, but it will ensure quality and consistency. Information on various manufacturers can be obtained from newsletters, websites, books, the Better Business Bureau, and your health care provider. For my own patients, I went through an exhaustive evaluation of several companies and now recommend a select handful. It is definitely worth the time and effort, as this can be a critical factor in the success or failure of your approach.

Progesterone Cream

The use of natural progesterone is another popular approach to treating PMS. The use of this regimen waxes and wanes. The utilization of progesterone for PMS is not new. In fact, it was one of the first "therapies" prescribed in an attempt to alleviate PMS symptoms. Dr. Katarina Dalton in the United Kingdom has long been an advocate for progesterone in the treatment of PMS. She has written extensively on the subject and remains, along with Dr. John Lee, one of progesterone's greatest advocates.

The use of progesterone for PMS is based on the theory that many of the PMS symptoms are due to progesterone deficiencies during the luteal phase of the cycle. This has subsequently been questioned; however, much attention is still being given to progesterone as a therapy.

Before we go any further, let's take a minute for a brief biochemistry lesson. It is easy to get confused with the terminology surrounding progesterone, so I want to clarify certain terms. The term *progesterone* identifies a specific molecule, a single substance. The term *progestin* refers to any substance that has progesterone-like action. For example, the commonly-used synthetic drug Provera (medroxyprogesterone acetate) is a progestin and not progesterone. It has some progesterone-like action, but because it is not the same substance it can have vastly different effects. The substances I will be referring to as "natural progesterone" are substances that are derived from plant sources and are exactly the same molecule that exists in your body.

The studies that have evaluated progesterone and PMS have had mixed results. A few have shown no beneficial effects while others have shown an improvement of symptoms over and above placebo. I suspect that this ambiguity is again due to the multifactorial nature of PMS. In my own practice I have used the natural progesterone cream with success in some women. I prefer a cream with a concentration of at least 400 mg of progesterone an ounce. It works best when used only during the luteal phase of the cycle at a starting dosage of 1/4-1/2 teaspoon rubbed on the abdomen or buttocks twice a day. This dose will deliver about 20-30 mg of progesterone a day. Note that this is a starting dose and almost always has to be adjusted depending on a woman's individual needs. A salivary test for free progesterone is especially helpful in monitoring progesterone absorption and levels during treatment.

This will not work for everyone; however, I have seen enough success in my practice that I feel it is an attractive alternative for some women. I will discuss progesterone cream in much more detail in the chapter on menopause.

Other Options

Several other herbal medicines have been associated with PMS treatment. These include Shepherd's Purse (Capsella Bursa Pastoris), Cyclamen (Cyclomen Europaeum), Bugleweed (Lycopus Virginicus), and Evening Primrose oil (Oenothera Biennis). I cannot recommend their use since no acceptable studies have been done to verify their effectiveness.

Patients have asked me about Homeopathy and PMS. Homeopathy is a system of healing originated in the early 1800s by Samuel Hahnemann, a German physician. It is based on the "doctrine of similars." In a nutshell, homeopaths believe that a substance that causes a symptom in a healthy person can be labeled a "remedy" and used to treat the same symptom in a sick person. They use extremely dilute mixtures of these "remedies" to treat a wide spectrum of illnesses. I am not trained in Homeopathy and my research and exposure to this field is limited, so I cannot recommend its use in either a positive or negative way. The benefit in trying a homeopathic treatment is that the solutions and capsules are so dilute the specter of adverse side effects is almost nonexistent.

Prescription Drugs

It is well-established that there are a variety of prescription medications available today for the treatment of PMS. Some of the most studied and successful are the family of medicines known as the serotonin re-uptake inhibitors. These include such well-known drugs as Prozac, Paxil, and Zoloft. They work by making available more of the neurohormone serotonin (the brain hormone that controls moods and emotions). There is an intimate association between depression, PMS, and various other emotional problems. The tie that binds is serotonin. These medicines are used primarily to treat depression; however, their utility in PMS is well-known. Several recent studies have shown a 70-75 percent improvement in PMS symptoms in women who take the medications either daily or just during the luteal phase of the cycle. In scientific studies there is a consistency of results with these medicines. In other words, they work more often than not!

However, not all is hunky-dory in Prozac land. All of these medications have significant side effects that often limit their use and effectiveness. As in any situation, with any medication, you have to weigh the good with the bad. My own bias is that these drugs are an absolute last resort for those who have made an honest and committed effort in other ways and still have significant, life-altering symptoms.

A great deal of PMS research is being devoted to a group of medicines known as the gonadotropin-releasing hormone agonists (GNRH agonist). They help reduce PMS, yet this is a clear case of the treat-ment being worse than the disease. The GNRH agonists induce a pseudo-menopause state and have a myriad of side effects. I have yet to see anyone who could not be helped significantly with other options without resorting to these harsh medications.

Summary

PMS is real! It is a medical entity that is defined by a spectrum of symptoms that can be both physical and emotional. It may intensify in the early to mid-forties and is sometimes confused with perimenopausal changes. The diagnosis is based on recurrent, repetitive symptoms mainly in the luteal phase of the cycle that are bothersome to the individual. Many factors influence symptoms, such as stress, nutrition, and activity level. The most critical step in treating PMS is making the proper diagnosis.

God has provided all the tools through nature and nurture to successfully attack PMS. The treatment of PMS symptoms consists of a step-by-step approach, that includes diet, exercise, lifestyle changes, and various vitamins and herbs.

Increasing the consumption of low-fat, high-fiber foods and avoiding excessive salt, caffeine and alcohol provide the framework for initial dietary changes. Converting to a vegetarian diet is a good long-term goal. Two major lifestyle adjustments that are mandatory in the successful treatment of PMS are adequate aerobic exercise and stress management.

Various "potions" are available to complement your dietary and lifestyle changes. Licorice root, black cohosh, chasteberry extract, and natural progesterone are but a few. Vitamins and minerals are also important. Vitamin E and B6, along with magnesium, calcium, and zinc, all have a special role in PMS therapy.

Remember you are "fearfully and wonderfully made," and God meets every need, whether it is health related or not. You have choices. So choose wisely.

Action Challenge

Pick one vitamin and herbal approach discussed, and apply it consistently for three months. (Continue to keep your symptom diary.) Shake your boody, literally, to the nearest herbal store and start today. Combine this with exercise, stress management, and a prayerful lifestyle and you will control PMS; it will not control you!

SECTION THREE

Is It Mental Pause or Menopause?

CHAPTER FIVE

The Perimenopause: The Forgotten Years

A wise person once said, "The only thing you can count on is that you can't count on anything!" This may be construed as a pessimistic viewpoint; however, it all depends on your perspective. Change is the one absolute in the world. Not a day goes by when you are not faced with changes. Some, in fact, most are minor changes. Yet there are times when the changes may be catastrophic. There are good changes, and there are bad changes. The critical question that must be answered every day is: "How are you going to deal with both the little and the not-so-little changes?" President Jimmy Carter said, "What is life if not adjustment–to different times, to our changing circumstances, and to each other?"

The midlife and the menopause are defined by change. In fact, when we capitalize the words "The Change," most adults know immediately about what we refer. Menopause is the "mother of all change."

To fully comprehend the nature of this "change," you must examine the time known as the perimenopause. This includes the months or years surrounding the menopause. It is the dress rehearsal for the big show. Some refer to this time as the climacteric, or premenopause. I prefer "perimenopause" because this is a more accurate characterization of the sequence of events. Besides, "climacteric" sounds funny to me and everyone has trouble pronouncing it!

Times, They Are a Changing

The perimenopause represents the months to years that surround the menopause. Remember that menopause is defined as the cessation of the periods. The average age for menopause in the United States is fifty-one. The perimenopause encompasses all of the events that go on before the periods cease. This time frame is different for every woman. Not everyone will experience "symptoms." The majority of women will sail through this time unencumbered by the shifting winds of change.

There is a great misperception that all women have signs and bothersome symptoms in the years leading up to and beyond menopause. It just doesn't happen that way. Those who have problems are just more vocal and visible than those who don't. You don't often hear from the 20–35 percent who don't experience hot flashes. I suspect, however, there are many women who have bothersome changes but elect not to discuss them at the office or the PTA. Anyway, the onset of the perimenopause is often subtle and in most cases identified only in retrospect. It is only after the fact that many realize, "Hey, all of these things I am experiencing may be related." There is no set age for the perimenopause just as there is no set age for menopause. Also, there is no set duration. It may last for six months or five years.

Am I There or What?

How do I know if I am perimenopausal? I usually answer patients who ask this with a series of questions: What is going on with you now? Are your periods regular? Are you experiencing hot flashes? Have you noticed a decreased sex drive? Are you fatigued? Do you have vaginal dryness? In other words, if you are experiencing symptoms of declining ovarian function, but are still having periods, you are perimenopausal.

What are some of these symptoms? Table 5 shows a partial list of symptoms that have been attributed to declining ovarian function. Don't let this list depress you; remember you may not experience any of these symptoms. Realize that God is not punishing you for growing older. A recent Gallup poll showed that more than 51 percent of perimenopausal/postmenopausal women felt that their life was better now (in the menopause) than it was before, and a majority of women believed that these feelings would continue.

TABLE 5
SYMPTOMS

Hot flashes	Irritability
Vaginal atrophy	Hair growth
Vaginal dryness	Low back pain
Vaginal burning	Vulvar itching
Vaginal itching	Bloating
Vaginal bleeding	Flatulence
Painful intercourse	Indigestion
Urinary incontinence	Osteoporosis
Urinary frequency	Deep bone ache
Urinary urgency	Thinning scalp hair
Painful urination	Breast tenderness
Depressed mood	Palpitations
Difficulty sleeping	Dizzy spells
Decreased libido	Headaches
Fatigue	"Crawly" skin
Impaired memory	Vertigo
Problems concentrating	Vaginal odor
Mood swings	Night sweats

It is empowering to educate yourself about what symptoms are associated with hormonal changes. The trap to avoid is associating *everything* that goes on at this time with hormonal changes. Establishing proper cause and effect between hormones and symptoms is a critical first step in alleviating those symptoms. There is a great deal of crossover in symptoms with other conditions, so be careful not to wear hormonal blinders.

Most symptoms will begin, if at all, during this perimenopausal time. So the operative word here is change. Your body is changing, your emotions are changing, and your environment is changing. Let's begin learning how to take charge and make this change a celebration. The first step is understanding the physical changes that begin the process.

Biology 101

The female reproductive system is a miraculous creation. It is a complex, integrated, perfectly-designed collection of organs, hormones, and tissues. There is no better example of how you are "wonderfully and fearfully made." The intricate interaction of all its parts overshadows any man-made creation.

The reproductive/endocrine system can be thought of as a three-story house. On the top floor sits the pituitary gland. This marble-sized structure at the base of the brain acts as the controller of the system. It sends out hormonal signals to the second story, the ovaries, and tells them to grow follicles that contain eggs. These developing follicles eventually respond to the pituitary's signals to stimulate ovulation. The ovaries, in addition to supporting and nourishing the developing eggs, secrete several hormones of their own, mainly estrogen, progesterone, and testosterone. The estrogen and progesterone act on the first story, the uterus, and lead to the buildup of the uterine lining and its eventual shedding, which is the monthly period. This cycle is repeated every 28–32 days unless one of the eggs that are shot out of the ovary meets up with a friendly sperm. If it is love at first sight, then the fertilized egg sets up a chain of events that leads to the uterine lining saying, "Hey, come on in and stay awhile—nine months to be exact."

As you age, the number of follicles in the ovary capable of developing into viable eggs decreases. At birth a woman has the greatest number of follicles she will ever possess. As the number of available follicles decreases there is a concurrent decrease in active ovulations. These cycles are called anovulatory cycles, and they are significant because they can lead to missed or irregular periods.

A balance between estrogen and progesterone is required for the normal development and subsequent shedding of the uterine lining. Ovulation is the regulator of this balance. If ovulation stops, then the normal cycle is disrupted. This is basically what happens in the perimenopause. The ovaries are ovulating less and less and this leads to a disruption of the normal cycles, and in turn to a change in the hormone production of both estrogen and progesterone. As the estrogen levels decrease, there is no stimulation for the uterine lining to grow. So there comes a point where the periods cease. Presto, menopause!

These changes don't happen overnight. I'll never forget a scene in the '70s TV show *All in the Family*. Edith is going through "the change," and Archie is becoming quite frustrated with the hot flashes and the moodiness. At one point he grabs Edith and throws her in a chair and says, "OK, Edith, you have exactly three minutes to get over this menopause thing!" It doesn't happen that way. These are slow processes that often occur over months or years. That is why the perimenopause is such a nebulous term with no set guidelines for duration; each woman is different.

When Will It Happen for Me?

Menopause is unique for every woman. You may experience four to five years of perimenopausal changes, whereas Aunt Mary may have one hot flash and stop her periods all within one month.

There does seem to be a genetic preprogramming built into the ovaries that instructs them when to begin to decrease their production of hormones. The only thing that has been even remotely associated with predicting when a particular woman may enter menopause is the age of her mother's menopause, and even that is a loose association.

There are many factors that may alter this onset. For example, women who smoke are noted to have earlier menopause than nonsmokers do. Women who have had a hysterectomy (but their ovaries were left in) tend to have an earlier menopause than they normally would have, but not by much.

So the perimenopause is, first and foremost, a time of change that is delineated by the onset of symptoms that are associated with declining hormone levels. It is appropriate to look at the idea of change and how to wrestle with it, because how you deal with change will influence your midlife experience. It should come as no surprise that the Bible has a great deal of wisdom to impart on this important topic.

A Real Life Scenario

Mary was a CEO of a startup software company. She was forty-five years old and had three children. Her husband worked in the same field, but with a different company. Mary came in for her yearly Pap smear and physical and told this story.

"Things have been really great this year. My company has finally seen some success, and I am beginning to really believe I am doing the right thing. Oh, sure, it has been incredibly stressful, but I feel like I am handling it well. I have noticed my periods have become a little more irregular, and I have actually skipped a few. The only thing that really bothers me is these stupid hot flashes. I can be making a presentation to a perspective client, and then all of a sudden, whoosh! I get red-faced and I break out in a sweat. I can only imagine what my client thinks. And I really believe I have lost an account or two because these flashes interrupted my presentation and broke my concentration.

"And that reminds me, I have noticed that I feel a little more forgetful these days. Not anything big, like where I am, but little things like where I put a paper or what I came into the room to get. It is not bad, but it does get annoying. I guess it's all a part of getting older, which is something I don't like at all!" Mary hesitated, and then continued. "If you get right down to it, what I don't like is this sense of not having complete control over my body and emotions. This is not me. I have always been able to handle about anything that comes along, but now at times I feel less able to do that, and it bothers me. Again, none of these things are really traumatic, but they do bother me, and I just am not sure how to deal with them in my life right now. I don't have time for these changes!"

Mary's story is a common one in the perimenopause. She has noticed some subtle changes in her body and emotions. These changes are not major or life-altering, yet they are noticeable and cause Mary to think about the future. One of the biggest fears of women in the perimenopause is losing control of their bodies and emotions. This is a disturbing feeling for many women that often prompts them to seek help or advice. Many, however, will not acknowledge they are troubled by this, and limit their options by ignoring the problem. It doesn't just go away by itself.

How do you deal with change? When faced with the inevitable changes brought on by aging, do you celebrate them or suffer by them? Do you confront the changes, or do you hide from them? Do you say, "I can handle this"? Or do you become an ostrich and bury your head in the sand?

The Bible teaches us how to deal effectively with change. God is unchanging and reliable. In the midst of chaos, confusion, and change, God and His love are constants. Those who have trouble with change are often seeking some form of stability, something solid and unchanging to grab onto to ride out the storm. Psalm 59:9–10 says, "You are my strength; I wait for you to rescue me, for you, O God, are my place of safety. In His unfailing love, my God will come and help me. He will let me look down in triumph on all my enemies."

Those are comforting words when things are exploding, as they sometimes seem to be at this time. Paul, talking of worries, tells us in Hebrews that God "will roll them up like an old coat. They will fade away like old clothing. But you are always the same; you will never grow old." (Hebrews 1:12)

Whenever you feel that the world around you is confusing and changing too fast, you can always find refuge in the stability and constancy of God and His Word. What is found in the Scripture is ageless and is the steady ship in the turbulent seas of the perimenopause.

One of the biggest problems with change is the lack of a constant basis for making decisions and judgments. Faced with change, we often call into question the values and beliefs we have relied upon in the past. For example, many women who notice mild depressive symptoms during the perimenopausal years often question their ability to "get over it" as they had done in the past. They had always been able to "pull themselves up by their bootstraps" and move on. It scares them when that doesn't work now. Things are changing. Accept the reality, but with every door that closes, another one opens. The buzzword for this time frame is adaptability.

The most important thing to keep in mind when you feel in this predicament is that there is a steady foundation you can rely on. There are beliefs and doctrines that can serve as beacons of light in an otherwise dark ocean of doubt. "Jesus Christ is the same yesterday, today, and forever" (Heb. 13:8). Here is your rock, your foundation, and your constant through these changing times.

"Heaven and earth will disappear, but my words will remain forever"(Mark 13:28).

Part of the Design

Remember that these changes are *of God*. These things are not independent of God. They don't exist in a vacuum. God does not leave you hanging over the abyss of hot flashes with nowhere to turn. You are never alone. In the midst of change, in the foggiest confusion... God is there. The answers and directions are there. "Praise the name of God forever and ever, for He alone has all wisdom and power. He determines the course of world events; He removes kings and sets others on the throne. He gives wisdom to the wise, and knowledge to the scholars." (Dan. 2:20–21)

It may be difficult to see God in the turbulence and discord that may occur in midlife. This can be a time when basic values are questioned, a time when a woman can believe that she is out of control. Many women feel they are "falling apart" and don't understand why. Many are comforted in knowing that all things are of God, even when times are hard-especially when times are hard! "And we know that God causes everything to work together for the good of those who love God and are called according to his purpose for them" (Rom. 8:28).

The perimenopause is a time of change. The first step in dealing with that change is the realization that God is in control and that there is a plan for you. But don't fall into the trap of thinking that since God is in control you can sit back, relax, and do nothing. You have to be an active participant in working through change. You are not a puppet of God. Free will and choice imply responsibility. This understanding allows you the freedom to face hardships and challenges with the comfort of a firm and unchanging foundation. At the outset, acknowledge that God is all-powerful and wants the best for you. You are subject to the natural laws of aging; however, if you apply the knowledge that God has provided, you can live in the midst of these changes joyously and abundantly.

Practical Ways to Handle Change

What are some practical ways to deal more effectively with change? Some of the suggestions that follow may sound simplistic, but I challenge you to actually do what I describe, and I know you will see a difference. Remember, if you keep doing things the same way, you will get the same result. If you are not happy with the result, you have to do something different, no matter how simple. I have found the most obvious suggestions are the ones we most likely ignore, and they can be the most effective. Knowledge is power, but the application of knowledge is wisdom. I read once where only 10 percent of people who order self-improvement tapes or "how to" tapes actually follow through with the ideas presented. I know I am guilty of good intentions on occasion, but good intentions never solved a single problem or relieved a single hot flash.

Here are fourteen ideas for handling change. Practice these simple suggestions daily and if you are not seeing results in a month, then I will . . . hmm, let me think on that one! As the Nike commercial says, "Just do it!"

Balance Work with Play

Schedule time for recreation. That doesn't mean jogging while listening to a tape of the latest stock quotes if you are a stockbroker. That means taking some time to *just be*. You don't have to do anything you don't want to do. We live in a hurry-up culture where it is important to always be accomplishing something. Busyness has become a virtue. That is not healthy. Certainly there is a place for goal setting and industrious behavior, but there is also a place for rest and play. Often our best decisions and perspectives come while at play. "That man is richest whose pleasures are the cheapest," said Henry David Thoreau.

Loaf a Little

Loaf a little. This is similar to number one, but mainly directed at those who need permission to do nothing. Do everything in moderation. This is not permission to become a couch potato but it is OK, dare I say even mandatory, to occasionally do nothing. It clears the mind and makes you more receptive to dealing with change. How can you do nothing? Be quiet, listen, nap, meditate, walk, run, daydream, or vegetate. Heed this prescription: Loaf five minutes,three times a day! Doctor's orders! "For God gives rest to his loved ones" (Ps. 127:2).

Get Adequate Sleep

Get enough sleep and rest. Simple. You have been berated with this continuously, yet that's because it is important! Waking and feeling refreshed is an indication that you are getting enough rest. One author recently went as far to say that if you use an alarm clock to wake you every morning, you are not getting enough rest. That may be taking things a bit far. I'm guilty myself. As a physician "on call" and a parent of two small children, I know about sleep deprivation. The problems often mimic those of menopause: poor concentration, forgetfulness, and irritability. On the seventh day God rested, and if it is OK for the Big Guy, it's OK for you.

Work off Tensions

Work off tensions. Physical exercise in any form—gardening, walking, cleaning house, working in the yard, or running the Boston Marathon—is an excellent way to work off irritating, angry, or depressed feelings. We will see in Chapter 7 that exercise is a scientifically-proven antidepressant. God created us to move, and exercise serves many purposes. Don't get your exercise by running your mouth, jumping to conclusions, being hopping mad, laying down the law, or hitting the wall!

Talk out Your Troubles

Talk out your troubles. Get things off your chest by talking with a sympathetic friend or family member. The fastest-growing "support groups" in this country are menopausal support groups. Talking with others experiencing the same tribulations not only reinforces that you are not crazy or alone, but it also provides helpful coping strategies. Part of this means being a good listener. Communication works best in a dialogue and not a monologue. God gave you two ears and one mouth so you would listen twice as much as you speak!

Don't forget about prayer. Taking your problems to God should be your first priority. You aren't reminding God of your struggles. He knows them. You are reminding yourself of your dependence on God. Don't forget to listen.

Get Away from It All

Get away from it all. Whether it is for an hour or a weekend, you need that time to regroup and think. A simple change of scenery may allow you enough time from the everyday stresses to gain new perspectives. I know many couples who have a specific date night (my wife and I included). We guard it carefully, because we know we need that time to reconnect with each other with no other distractions. It says to both of us, "You are important, and I cherish the time we have alone together." My wife sometimes gets upset with me when I turn down social invitations on our date night, because she enjoys those much more than I do. However, she also understands that my need to "get away from it all" includes social obligations, and I jealously guard our time alone together.

Some people need time to be truly alone, by themselves. It is OK to say to a spouse or child, "I need some quiet time so I can be a better me." This is not selfish or aloof behavior, for if you can come back refreshed and rejuvenated, you can be a much better spouse, parent, or friend. This does not mean abandoning your responsibilities and commitments to "find yourself." This is a time (whether for ten minutes or a week), to reestablish your connection to God and to reaffirm your life's direction.

The Bible is full of examples of people who "got away from it all" and came back full of the Spirit of God. Moses spent a lot of time on the mountain in prayer and meditation. The apostle Paul spent several years of contemplation after his conversion experience before he began his ministry. Jesus went into the garden alone to pray before his capture and crucifixion.

Avoid Self-Medication

Avoid self-medication. Alcohol is one of the most dangerous medications in times of stress and change. The temptation is to dull the anxiety. The reality is you need to be at your best, physically and mentally, to positively and permanently handle change. You can't do this if you are loaded! As the prophet Hosea laments, "Alcohol and prostitution have robbed my people of their brains" (Hosea 4:11). Croft Pentz once said, "Many things can be preserved in alcohol, but Christian character is not one of them."

Be Proactive with Your Health

Be proactive with your health. This is a message that I preach throughout this book. Do not wait for an illness to hit before you take action. Prevention is paramount. Studies have shown that people in stressful, times or undergoing massive change in their lives are more susceptible to illness. Anticipate this and take steps to reduce that likelihood by getting proper rest, eating as I have suggested, and using various herbs, vitamins, and nutritional supplements. I am seeing a healthy shift in many women's approach to menopause. They are taking steps to preempt problems instead of reacting to them. This applies to handling change also-anticipate and react. Seek the advice and counsel of those who have dealt with change effectively. "Plans go wrong for lack of advice; many counselors bring success"(Prov. 15:22).

Take One Thing at a Time

Take one thing at a time. Schedule your work so that you can concentrate solely on one thing. Don't waste your time by fretting over how much you have to do. Do something! The key here is focus. Pour your energies into completing one task before you launch into another. There is only a small difference between schizophrenia and normal thinking. Many experts feel it is a problem of focus. Somehow the brain disconnects the normal pathways and ideas and thoughts become jumbled. The ability to focus on a task is crucial in being able to complete it.

Change can create a sense of being overwhelmed. Take each problem or situation one at a time, focusing on solving that one task before tackling the next. Every thousand-mile journey begins with the first step. My wife is a great list-maker. She gets satisfaction by making lists, and then, with great fanfare, scratching each item off as it is accomplished. This keeps her focused and helps to ward off the feelings of "I'll never get this done."

Avoid Superwoman Syndrome

Be careful of the superwoman syndrome. This is especially important to women with career and family responsibilities. You can't do everything, and you can't do everything perfectly. Divide duties, delegate responsibilities, and concentrate on what you can do best. This caution is new because the majority of the households in the United States are now two-income families. The expectations of others (and yourself) can be unrealistic. The choice is one of priorities.

Steven Pollan, in his book *Living Rich*, describes work as a tool only for making money. He asserts that your job cannot and should not serve as emotional or spiritual fulfillment. It is good to like what you do, but the bottom line is that it makes you money. He says how you feel about the work is largely irrelevant. I don't agree with much of what he says, but I do believe that too often we try to find satisfaction, identity and meaning on the job, often at the exclusion of home and family. Your work can be a spiritual path, yet trying to find inner peace on the job can lead you down a deceptive road.

Set life priorities, and then make decisions about work, home, church, and family that align with those priorities. If trying to be superwoman is getting you down, prioritize. Eliminate those activities and responsibilities that don't fit in your priority list. Stream-line, sit back, and simplify. H. Norman Wright says in his book *Simplify Your Life and Get More Out of It*, "We honestly believe that life can no longer be simple. But it can. It's not just an illusion. It's within reach. But this means risking, changing and taking a close look at . . . you!"[1] This simplification cannot be piecemeal, however. It may involve a complete spring cleaning from the inside out! In Mark 2:21–22, Jesus said, "And who would patch an old garment with unshrunk cloth? For the new patch shrinks and pulls away from the old cloth, leaving an even bigger hole than before. And no one puts new wine into old wineskins. The wine would burst the wineskins, spilling the wine and ruining the skins. New wine needs new wineskins."

Do for Others

Do something for others. Escape from the preoccupation with yourself by lending a helping hand to those in need. We are here to serve, and nothing helps a person effectively handle change than by doing something meaningful for someone else. The best place to find a helping hand is at the end of your own arm. To feel sorry for the needy is not the mark of a Christian—to help them is.

Set Realistic Goals

Set realistic goals. Goals are important. Most successful people actually have a set of written goals lying around somewhere. A study done of Harvard graduates that were followed for twenty years showed that the people who were most accomplished in their respective fields were those who had written goals. The secret is to at least think about what you want to accomplish. There is nothing wrong with lofty goals, but they do have to be achievable. For example, it would be rather unrealistic for me to set a goal of running a twenty six mile marathon in two and a half hours (I can't even *drive* twenty-six miles in that time). A much more realistic, yet still challenging goal would be to run a three-and-a-half hour marathon. Don't set yourself up for failure by setting unrealistically high goals and expectations. Hans Christian Andersen said, "Nothing is too high for a man to reach, but he must climb with care and confidence."

Some of us may set our goals too low, (or not have specific goals at all) so we must be realistic too. There are some things beyond our reach, but not so many as we think. Our goals should be high enough to challenge us, high enough that we climb with care and confidence, but not so high that they are impossible to reach.

Make and Use Lists

If you are having trouble concentrating, keep lists and use them. A certain degree of organization is helpful during any transition. Because of the innate chaos of change, having written lists of tasks gives you something concrete to focus on. It is like a lighthouse in the fog, pointing you to a safe harbor. Balance is important here. Don't be obsessive about it and make lists of your lists!

Slow Down

Slow down. Give yourself permission to listen to your body. Ease up on yourself when the hormones won't. We live in a fast-paced, hurry-up world. My wife is fond of saying she wants this done and done yesterday! The only person who can slow down the process of change is you. You do this by consciously knowing from where the change originates and pulling in the reins. Change is inevitable, but you can have some control over the pace.

Laurie Beth Jones talks about "energy leaks" in her book *Jesus CEO*. Energy was something Jesus was acutely aware of. You remember the story of the woman in the crowd who suffered from a bleeding problem. She knew that if she was able to touch Jesus she would be healed. At the moment she touched His garment, He felt the healing energy leave him. "But Jesus told him, `No, someone deliberately touched me, for I felt healing power go out from me'" (Luke 8:46). Laurie Beth Jones goes on to say, "How many energy leaks do we have in our own daily lives? Leaks such as angry words, distractions, or tampering in someone else's business while neglecting our own. Energy is everywhere, but stillness plays a major role in conversion from "potential" to "actualized" energy."[2] You control the flow of energy thereby controlling the flow of change. Slow down.

You may look at these suggestions and say that they sound, too simple or not profound enough However I can tell you, from watching and working with hundreds of women in the perimenopause, that they will work if you consistently and honestly apply them. Taking action is the key. Knowing all of this is worthless unless it becomes applied knowledge. Jesus knew the benefit of taking action. When he was chastised by the Pharisees for healing on the Sabbath, he responded, "My Father never stops working, so why should I?" (John 5:17) Jesus knew the importance of doing!

Life Balance

The stress of the perimenopause and other life changes impacts each woman differently. One of the ways to master the physical and psychological challenges of this transition is to be acutely aware of your internal signals. This is a matter of focusing on what you are thinking and feeling and trying to distinguish whether it is hormone related or not. This is where a trained, knowledgeable health care worker can be invaluable. A helpful technique is to keep a diary of physical and emotional symptoms and discuss them with your friend and ally in this transition. As in PMS, an accurate record of what symptoms are present and how they affect you can be an invaluable tool to both you and your doctor. Keeping a written record helps you to understand and identify feelings and how they influence your actions.

I want to introduce a term called "life balance". This is an important concept during change, because it forces you to analyze feelings and experiences and to discover facets of your life that need balance. I've talked about the importance of balance before in dealing with health. Health is a state of balance among mind, body, and spirit. Life balance can be applied daily, and it acts as a stabilizing refuge in the winds of change.

When you are in control of your life, you are able to give an appropriate amount of time and energy to those things that are important to you. Balance allows women to feel a sense of contentment in meeting the demands of life.

When you are in life balance, you feel it. You are energetic, physically healthy, optimistic, and in control. Others can observe it in your behavior. You don't come unglued at the least little thing. You are even-tempered, you feel good, and you get along with others. When you can dissipate negative feelings from a stressful day before starting a new day, you are in balance.

When you are out of life balance, others may hint that you are acting out of sorts or seem to be in a perpetual bad mood. Often you feel a vague sense of discomfort, that "I can't pinpoint it but I know something is wrong" feeling. Some specific signs of imbalance are fatigue, vague discontent, sense of helplessness or hopelessness, anxiety or guilt, low self-esteem, inability to make decisions, and difficulty in focusing on a task.

People who are out of balance may abuse their bodies through alcohol, smoking, and doing little or no exercise. They may have low energy and motivation, be impatient and critical, and become annoyed, especially when others place demands on them. Recognize that you are not alone if you experience these problems. In a recent survey of over 25,000 perimenopausal women in the United States, a majority of women confessed that at times they felt out of control and experienced these symptoms.

You may be asking, "What does all this have to do with menopause?" We talked earlier of all the symptoms of the perimenopause. The signs and symptoms of imbalance and the signs and symptoms of menopause are similar. Behavioral medicine recognizes that the mind and body are intimately connected and the two cannot be separated. God has also shown the two are interdependent in His writings, long before behavioral medicine "discovered" this association. "You must love the Lord your God with all your heart, all your soul, and all your mind" (Matt. 22:37). This illustrates that each of us has an important role in our own well-being. Being in life balance allows us the ability to blossom. One approach to achieving balance is through a concept called self-efficacy.

Self-Efficacy

Self-efficacy is a belief in your ability to exercise control over specific events in your life. Dr. Albert Bandura at Stanford University Medical School has shown that a strong sense of self-efficacy is the best and most consistent predictor of positive health outcomes in many different situations. In other words, you feel that you can control the event (change) instead of the event (change) controlling you. In reality what you are controlling is your perception of and reaction to the event.

If you live long enough, you will experience menopause. Those who have a strong sense of self-efficacy believe that they have control over how menopause will be experienced. In most cases, this becomes a self-fulfilling prophecy.

Life responsibilities are time-consuming, and we find ourselves occupied by the many demands of others and ourselves. It is easy to get caught up in the requests of others while our wants and needs become lost. If your life is to be in balance, you must know what is important to you, not what others think should be important to you. You must know your values, your strengths, your weaknesses, and your goals. Dr. Neal Warren, in his book *Finding Contentment*, states that true contentment now and at any time in life is achieved by being authentic. This is especially true in the perimenopause. He states, "You can experience enduring contentment only when you have the courage to be deeply and profoundly your true self, the self you discover when you make careful and solid choices about your life all along the way."[3]

If you believe that you can control those choices, that you can be the boss lady, then you will be able to achieve satisfaction in all aspects of your midlife experience.

The greatest benefit of the transition time is that it offers an opportunity to develop a future self, a new balance between output and input. For some women the decision to balance their lives means to cut down on work, to take on a new hobby, to start a new job, to go back to school, to climb a mountain, or to run a marathon. For others it involves changing unhealthy habits, stopping smoking, starting to exercise, and learning what their bodies need to feel good.

The optimistic belief that you are in control, capable, and competent to make changes in your life is important to health. Studies have shown that women who have a positive outlook and feel a sense of control experience fewer adverse symptoms of the perimenopause. The more clearly you visualize your ideal self, the more comfortable you will be with becoming that person.

There is help from the Bible. There are role models, as we will see in Naomi and other Bible women. I challenge you to balance your life with a foundation of prayer and the Word. Rejoice in the knowledge that God has provided women with the brain power and belief systems to be healthy, happy, and content.

Self-efficacy doesn't diminish our dependence on the sovereignty and power of God. It is about choices. God is the ultimate controller. As children of God we are given choices of paths to follow. Self-efficacy is about choosing a path that empowers and permits you to live the meaningful and joyous life that God intends.

Action Challenge

Reread the fourteen ways to handle change: Commit to learning and *practicing* three new strategies a week. You will feel remarkably better in a month.

CHAPTER SIX

Menopause: Puberty with Experience

The biggest problem with menopause is "brain drain." Some women need Roto Rooter for their attitude in dealing with menopause. Women are taught from early on (in this culture) that aging is not something to be cherished. Aging is often demonized and feared. In talks I give, I always play a word association game with the audience. When I say, "menopause," someone says "aging" (and that's one of the nicer things they say). For many, menopause is intimately linked to the idea of growing old, and this is inevitably and negative association.

You may be thinking that your have every right to associate menopause with negative feelings. With hot flashes every minute, skin dryer and Sahara, the sex drive of a coffee mug, and a husband who wants you to "get over it." your have a case for this not being the golden years you dreamed of! Ashleigh Brilliant said, "Inside every older person there is a younger person, wondering what happened!"[1]

Yet, if that approach has you where you don't want to be, then the obvious choice is to change your approach. What have you got to lose except your misery? Max Lucado puts it this way:

> Life has rawness and wonder. Pursue it. Hunt for it. Don't listen to the whines of those who have settled for a second rate life and want you to do the same. Your goal is not to live long; it is to live.
>
> You think staying inside is safe? Jesus disagrees. "Whoever seeks to save his life will lose it." Reclaim the curiosity of your childhood. Just because you are near the top of the hill doesn't mean you have passed your peak.[2]

This chapter outlines how you can change your attitude toward menopause. It's time to take the ovaries by the "horns" and come up with options and solutions. This is the cornerstone of a healthy approach: choice. We must give women the knowledge that allows them to prayerfully consider what is best for them.

In the pages of the Old Testament you find a wonderful role model for today's midlife woman. All the success gurus proclaim that modeling is one of the most effective methods of achieving success. Why reinvent the wheel? If you can find someone who has accomplished what you desire to achieve, use as a model, a mentor, and teacher. This commonly applies to a career, but can also be manifested in your day-to-day existence. God has provided the midlife woman with an excellent role model in the person of Naomi.

Ruth and Naomi

Benjamin Franklin was the ambassador to France in the early part of our country's existence. He was an occasional attendee of a group known as the Infidels Club, an arrogant group that spent its time researching and reading literary masterpieces. On one occasion when it was Ambassador Franklin's time to read, he chose to read the Book of Ruth, but he changed the names so it would not be recognized as a book of the Bible.

When he finished his reading the praise from the group was universal. They stated that it was one of the most beautiful and inspiring short stories they had ever heard, and they immediately wanted to know who was the author and where he had discovered such a magnificent literary masterpiece. He was overjoyed to tell them that it was from the Bible, which they had held in low regard for its literary and moral value.

The short book of Ruth gives us one of the greatest role models for the "mature" woman. Naomi was a Jewish woman who lived in Bethlehem with her husband, Elimelech, in the time of the judges. They had two sons, Mahlon and Chilion. As was often the case in their homeland, a famine hit the area of Bethlehem. Elimelech decided to move his family to the land of Moab, east of the Dead Sea, in search of more fertile land. Now Moab was a pagan nation that was the perpetual enemy of Israel, and Naomi and her family were foreigners in a hostile land.

Soon after they arrived, Elimelech died, leaving Naomi a widow with two sons. The sons married two Moabite women, Orpah and Ruth. In contrast to all future TV situation comedies, these women and their mother- in- law got along famously and built strong bonds. Ten years into their life in Moab, the two sons died. It is speculated that these two boys were not healthy, strapping physical specimens, as the son's names are translated "Weakness" and "Perishing." I can only imagine what was going through Elimelech's mind when he bestowed such loving names on his only sons.

So now Naomi is widowed and without her sons in a strange and sometimes hostile land, yet her daughters-in-law remain devoted to her. In fact, their bond only strengthens. Soon Naomi gets word that the famine in her homeland has ended, so she makes the logical decision to return home where her family had resided years earlier. There she hopes to find comfort and support. When she tells her daughters-in-law of her intentions, although she puts them under no obligation, they desire to return with her. Naomi beseeches them both to stay in their homeland to be with their immediate families. She desperately wants them to find new husbands and begin a new life. With great agony Naomi encourages the girls to stay in Moab, and tearfully, Orpah agrees.

However, Ruth steadfastly proclaims her loyalty and commitment to Naomi in this beautiful passage: "But Ruth replied, `Don't ask me to leave you and turn back. I will go wherever you go and live wherever you live. Your people will be my people, and your God will be my God. I will die where you die and will be buried there. May the LORD punish me severely if I allow anything but death to separate us!"(Ruth 1:17)

Naomi relents, and she and Ruth travel to Bethlehem and arrive just as the harvest is beginning. Naomi knows well the laws of the land, and she tells Ruth that she may go to the fields and "glean" (or gather up) any leftover grain after the harvesters have passed through the fields. This was a long-established custom spelled out in Leviticus 19:9: "When you harvest your crops, do not harvest the grain along the edges of your fields, and do not pick up what the harvesters drop. It is the same with your grape crop—do not strip every last bunch of grapes from the vines, and do not pick up the grapes that fall to the ground. Leave them for the poor and the foreigners who live among you, for I, the LORD, am your God."

God had made provisions for the poor and widowed. Ruth gleaned in the field of Boaz, a wealthy and respected landowner who was related to Naomi's dead husband, Elimelech. Ruth quickly learns that she has caught the eye of Boaz, a fact not lost on Naomi. As it becomes obvious that Boaz is showing Ruth special favor, Naomi begins formulating a plan to get them together. The months pass, and Ruth is the picture of proper and industrious behavior. She realizes that Boaz favors her, yet, on tutelage from Naomi, she makes no demands on him. Again in a brilliant use of the Levirate law, Naomi decides to put Elimelech's land up for sale. She knows that her dead husband's next of kin is required by law to buy the plot. She instructs Ruth in the proper way of letting Boaz know that she is interested in Boazs affections, and waits for her plan to unfold.

There is a hitch, however. Boaz tells Ruth of another man in town who is actually closer in kin to Elimelech, and by law he has the first right of refusal on the land. Boaz, a man used to getting what he wants, tells Ruth not to fret, he will think of something.

The scene then shifts to the city gates, which are like our town hall, where Boaz confronts the relative. He asks if he is prepared to buy the land, and when he says, "Yes," Boaz continues. He states that if the relative buys the land, then he must also marry Ruth. Boaz also states that it would be his duty to father a child so Elimelech's line would not die out. Implied in this, which is not lost on the relative, is that the land he just purchased would go to Ruth's child and would not be passed to his own offspring. So, in essence, he would be buying land that would never really be owned by him. Now remember this is not only about fulfilling the law but also, and I dare say more importantly, about economics. The relative is not so concerned about the marriage as he is about losing the land to Ruth's offspring. He ponders all this and finally states that he doesn't think this is a good thing and backs out of the deal.

This was the response that Boaz had counted on, so he immediately calls together the elders of the town and proclaims his intentions to buy the land, marry Ruth, and act as the "redeemer" for Elimelech's family.

After the marriage Ruth bears a son who was called Obed, which means "worship." Then, "Naomi took care of the baby and cared for him as if he were her own. The neighbor women said, `Now at last Naomi has a son again!" (Ruth 4:17) The story doesn't end there, as we are then told that Obed is the grandfather of the great King David, ancestor of Jesus.

This wonderful story goes much beyond being just an exciting and beautiful narrative. The person of Naomi serves as important role model for all midlife women. We know Naomi is in the perimenopause or perhaps the menopause as she states, "Can I still give birth to other sons who could grow up to be your husbands? No, my daughters, return to your parents' homes, for I am too old to marry again." She is past the age of childbearing and so will not remarry.

Naomi illustrates behaviors that are vital for living a healthy, happy, and meaningful life today. The magnificence of the Bible is in its timeliness. Its stories, characters, and wisdom are as applicable today as when they were first told by the elders around campfires.

Menopausal Roles

Naomi's story illustrates three areas of strength in a woman's character. She acts as a friend, a teacher, and a nurturer—three roles that a woman in the midlife is in a unique position to fulfill. These three roles are essential to the perpetuation of the wisdom of women and the bonds that tie generations together.

Friend

First and foremost, Naomi was a friend to Ruth. She illustrated the importance of friendship between women of different backgrounds and generations. She was family, not by blood, but by bond. This bond was made strong by friendship. Women in midlife have opportunities to form caring bonds with other women of similar and dissimilar backgrounds. They are bound by their experiences as women and their desire to communicate on a caring level. They are helped through difficult times by God's love and extraordinary devotion to one another. Just as Naomi was bolstered in tragic and extremely difficult times by the love and friendship of Ruth, so women today can gain great comfort and joy through their associations with other women.

Support groups, family members, health care professionals, and friends can all form a network of caring that can help a woman struggling with menopause. Reach out; seek other women who are experiencing similar problems. Make the effort. In a fabulous book called *Women of the Fourteenth Moon: Writings on Menopause*, women relate their experiences with menopause. These experiences range from the transcendent to the mundane. They illustrate that even though each woman's menopausal experience is unique, there is a common thread that ties women together, a mysterious bond that is only shared by those who have felt and experienced menopause—creating a dialogue among understanding friends. Naomi and Ruth exemplify that this bond can cross generations because friendship is ageless.

If Naomi were around today, I'm sure she would have been a founding member of the Widows from Moab support group! She knew the importance of friendship.

Naomi also illustrates how vital it is to remain faithful to God and His love through tough times. No one could argue that she had known heartache and sorrow. She, like Job, had lost loved ones, stature, and sustenance. She could have easily have lamented, "Why me?" and been justified in doing so. However, she models the way God can work through a woman who refuses to throw a pity party but instead chooses to move forward with life. Naomi doesn't wait for things to happen to her, she embraces life and creates opportunities. She knows that God has not abandoned her, and He has greater plans for her life.

How many times do we cry out when hard times come, not understanding and trusting in God that there is a greater meaning? Into Naomi's greatest darkness, after the death of her husband and two sons, God delivers Ruth, the beloved daughter-in-law who extends to Naomi her unconditional love. What an incredible support that must have been! This in turn empowers Naomi to go back into the day and make the rest of her life meaningful and joyous.

God can and will do this for you today through the living Christ. You have to acknowledge this and accept it as Naomi did. She could have rejected the affection of Ruth and forbidden her to return with her to Bethlehem. This, no doubt, would have led to a lifetime of misery and regret. As a woman in the menopause, you must understand that your present and future years will be infinitely more content if you accept the gift of faith and the belief that God has a plan for you even now. Naomi learned that, even in the middle of great suffering and sadness, God was full of mercy and goodness. Though your midlife experience may not be filled with as many adversities as Naomi (I hope not), the underlying message is the same.

Teacher

The second role that is important in defining a woman's experience in menopause is that of a teacher. Naomi acts as a mentor to Ruth in ways of love, economics, and religion. This idea of an older woman mentoring a younger woman has largely fallen by the wayside in today's society. It lies as another casualty in the death of the extended family. No longer do women have immediate access to older family members—sisters, mothers, grandmothers, or mothers-in-law.

Most commonly this situation arises from geographic separation; however, I believe it goes deeper than that. I sense from patients that there is an emotional separation that is much wider than any land mass. Lucky and fortunate is the woman who has a mentor to model wisdom and relay life experiences. And blessed is the older woman who can act as a guide in helping others navigate the treacherous waters of midlife. There is a tremendous benefit to both.

This emotional and geographic separation is a major problem for many women entering the menopause. Many have few to consult, collaborate, or communicate with. I can't tell you how many women come into my office totally in the dark about menopause, and explain that they have had no one to talk with about it. Time and time again I hear, "My mother never talked about it," or "I was not around much when this was going on so I don't know what to expect."

God did not design it this way. In the story of Ruth and Naomi, He shows that the proper education about this life event (or any life event) comes not from the streets or the media or even books, but from caring, knowledgeable, trusted women who have been there and done that! That is not to say that part of this education can't come from additional sources (for example, a well-written informaltive book). But there is no substitution for mentoring by one who cares about you. Most meaningful relationships are based on giving: giving love, time, attention, knowledge, and advice. The relationship between women in different life roles is also one of giving, and this connection flows in both directions. Both women involved in a mentoring relationship benefit immensely.

Notice that Naomi gives advice on many topics, including love (how to capture Boaz's affections), economics and law (the land purchase deal), and religion (Ruth took Naomi's God as her own). Virtually no important area of these women's lives was off-limits, because they were committed to each other's well-being.

I challenge you to seek out women to share in your experience and to discover those who would benefit from your wisdom. They may be right under your nose!

Nurturer

The third role that this narrative illustrates for the menopausal woman is that of nurturer. To nurture is to stimulate, encourage, challenge, and protect in a loving manner that allows the person to grow.

Naomi actually becomes a live-in grandmother at the end of the story. This is a role that many would cherish but few today get to experience. Again, the separation among families, both physically and emotionally, makes this difficult. We can only speculate on the interaction between Naomi and Obed, her grandson; however, it can be safely stated that Naomi's primary role was that of nurturer.

This role appears to benefit Naomi as much as it does Obed and Ruth. Look at the final few verses of the fourth chapter. "`May this child restore your youth and care for you in your old age. For he is the son of your daughter-in-law who loves you so much and who has been better to you than seven sons!' Naomi took care of the baby and cared for him as if he were her own. The neighbor women said, `Now at last Naomi has a son again!' And they named him Obed. He became the father of Jesse and the grandfather of David." So in this role as nurturer, the menopausal woman will not only find purpose, but will also reap the benefits of bestowing her care and wisdom on generations to come. It was through Naomi's love and attention that the lineage of Jesus Christ was preserved.

Action Challenge

Write down all the roles you have now: mother, grandmother, wife, friend, and so on. Then consider how valuable and unique each role is. Ponder how many people would be impacted if you didn't fill those roles. Understand your uniqueness in God's plan for not only you but the people around you.

CHAPTER SEVEN

The Four A's

Let me say again what I said at the beginning of this book: **Menopause is not a disease!** I know you may be questioning this after seeing all the potential symptoms and afflictions, yet always keep in mind that this is a normal, natural transition that may be punctuated by various physical or emotional changes.

I have a proven prescription for celebrating menopause. I have witnessed hundreds of women in the past eleven years make this a joyous celebration by living these simple suggestions. I have seen women experience not only the improvement of symptoms but also a deeper understanding of themselves and their bodies, and a closer tie to the Creator who designed them to be healthy.

The four-step prescription for making this time a joyous celebration is represented by the four A's I mentioned in Chapter 1: Attitude, Aptitude, Action, and Apothecary. These are like the four legs on a chair. They work best if they are all there and working equally. If one is cut short, balance is hard to achieve. Each area is important in its own right, and, together the harmony is magical.

ATTITUDE

Attitude is first because it is the foundation on which to build. "A relaxed attitude lengthens life; jealousy rots it away" (Prov.14:30).

We are what we believe. Our mindset is so incredibly powerful that it can dictate our reality. God has given us an unbelievably useful brain, if only we would use it more often. Paul's letter to the Romans says that what is in our hearts and minds is of the utmost importance. "For the Kingdom of God is not a matter of what we eat or drink, but of living a life of goodness and peace and joy in the Holy Spirit. If you serve Christ with this attitude, you will please God. And other people will approve of you, too." (Rom. 14:18)

Study after study has shown that a woman's perception of menopause markedly affects her experience. The old, worn idea of the self-fulfilling prophecy is still relevant because it is true. As you believe, so shall it be! A study a few years back compared the symptoms of menopausal women in Japan with those in America. When all confounding factors were eliminated (including the consumption of soy products) one of the greatest influences on the severity of symptoms was the belief system of the participants. In other words, the Japanese women, who had a much more positive approach to aging and menopause, had fewer symptoms in all categories. The U.S. women loathed and feared aging, and this had a marked impact on their symptom profile.

We touched on the importance of attitude in the chapter on PMS. It can't be stressed enough that viewing menopause as a time for growth, freedom, and excitement will alter your experience. Margaret Mead, anthropologist and author, described what she called the "postmenopausal zest." This was a realization that life is what we make it, a realization that God has a plan for all, even as we age, a realization that you are going to spend a third of your life in menopause—so it is not a time to pack it in and give up!

Charles Swindoll says, "Words can never adequately convey the incredible impact of our attitude toward life. The longer I live the more convinced I become that life is 10 percent what happens to us and 90 percent how we respond to it."[1] He also says,

> This may shock you, but I believe the single most significant decision I can make on a day-to-day basis is my choice of attitude. It is more important than my past, my education, my bankroll, my successes or failures, fame or pain, what other people think of me or say about me, my circumstances, or my position. Attitude is that "single string" that keeps me going or cripples my progress. It alone fuels my fire or assaults my hope. When my attitudes are right, there's no barrier too high, no valley too deep, no dream too extreme, no challenge too great for me.[2]

Where does this attitude come from? How do you get this attitude?

You practice! You start slowly, taking one thing at a time, and before long you notice that a transformation has taken place. In other words, identify one destructive belief and work on eliminating or changing it, and then move on to the next. The biggest reason people fail or have trouble starting the process is that they feel overwhelmed. They feel the task is either to frightening or too huge to achieve. By focusing on one problem at a time, you can end up altering your entire perspective.

Psychoneuroimmunology

The branch of science that studies how attitudes affect the body's immune system is known as psychoneuroimmunology. Multiple studies have shown that how we think, feel, and believe can markedly affect the functioning of the most basic building block of protection from disease, the white blood cell. Anger, anxiety, compassion, joy, and many other positive and negative emotions have been noted to alter the ability of white blood cells to ward off infection. Intuitively, scientists have known that people under a great deal of stress are more susceptible to illness; now many acknowledge this as the reason why. We have all been in situations where the stress level is exaggerated and know that if we are around anyone with a cold or flu, we will inevitably succumb.

When it comes to attitude, I challenge you to think abnormally. Just as I encouraged you to think abnormally about diet, I encourage you to develop an "abnormal" attitude. Normal is not necessarily healthy. "Thinking outside of the box" is a favorite corporate buzz phrase, and yet it applies to your beliefs and attitudes. Think abnormally in the sense of not following the crowd and not accepting what is "normal" as necessarily what is "right." Jesus certainly thought abnormally. He was a radical in his ideas and teachings. In fact it was this "abnormal thought" that proved to be his downfall in the eyes of the Jewish rulers, but the salvation of Christians the world over.

> In the movie *The Poseidon Adventure*, the ocean liner SS Poseidon is on the open sea when it hits a huge storm. Lights go out, smoke pours into rooms and, amid all the confusion, the ship flips over.
>
> Because of the air trapped inside the ocean liner, it floats upside down. But in the confusion, the passengers can't figure out what's going on. They scramble to get out, mostly by following the steps to the top deck. The problem is, the top deck is now 100 feet under water. In trying to get to the top of the ship, they drown.
>
> The only survivors are the few who do what doesn't make sense. They do the opposite of what everyone else is doing and climb up into the dark belly of the ship until they reach the hull. Rescuers hear them banging and cut them free.
>
> In life, it's as if God has turned the ship over and the only way for us to find freedom is to choose what doesn't make sense: live our lives by serving, supporting, and sacrificing for others.[3]

It Happens Every Day

Elisa was confused. She thought she was handling many of the changes of menopause effectively, yet she experienced one symptom that she couldn't get a grip on. She had no libido. Her sex drive had driven off. It had not always been that way. She and her husband, Roy, had enjoyed a healthy sex life through most of their twenty-two years of marriage. Elisa was fifty-one and her periods had stopped seven months earlier. She had experienced a few hot flashes, but that was about it as far as "the change" for her. When she came to see me she was concerned because this problem had begun to create friction in her marriage. We talked extensively about her prior feelings and what was different now.

What became obvious after several minutes of discussion was that Elisa held many irrational thoughts and myths about sexuality in the menopause. She had heard from her friends that it was natural to have a decreased libido as you age, and she believed this was "normal." Her husband did not share this belief. She also thought that, as she aged, she was becoming less physically attractive to her husband. She had gained about six pounds over the past year, and she was embarrassed by the shift in her center of gravity. She reported that she had noticed some decreased lubrication during sex, but said she thought that was "par for the course." When questioned further, Elisa did admit that the few times she had sex over the past several months it had been physically uncomfortable.

The first step in solving Elisa's dilemma was to eliminate the myths and provide accurate information, essentially changing her attitude. Studies have shown absolutely no correlation between sex drive and age. Many women in my practice report an active sex life well into their later years. A recent study in the *Journal of the American Medical Association* reports that women over fifty actually have fewer sexual problems than those under fifty.

I will never forget the little old lady who was having difficulty remembering to take her hormones on time. She was seventy-six. I thought I needed to give her some help in remembering, so I suggested that she associate taking her hormones with a common task she did automatically every day. I think I used the example of brushing her teeth or something similar. She came back two months later and said, "Dr. Eaker, your suggestion worked beautifully. I haven't missed a pill since I started taking them after my husband and I make love."

My initial reaction was, Oh no! She must have misunderstood me, and I explained to her that the pills were supposed to be taken every day.

She just smiled and said, "Yes, I know!"

Second, Elisa and I explored the idea that sexual intimacy is much more than physical attractiveness. Her looks were changing, but her heart and soul was still the woman Roy loved. She knew this on a cognitive level, but just needed to have it restated in the proper emotional context.

Third, I made sure she understood the link between aging, declining estrogen, and vaginal lubrication. Many women do experience dryness in the menopause that arises from decreased secretion of the vaginal glands. This can lead to pain and discomfort with intercourse. Consciously or unconsciously, if it hurts, you don't want to do it! The good news is that for this and other problems of menopause there are many solutions.

The resolution of Elisa's problem began with an attitude change. She began to understand the complex nature of the sex drive and discarded the belief that sex was not for the older generation. She changed the way she viewed her own sexuality and embraced the options available to her to counteract her physical problems.

Prayer

Another effective way to orchestrate an attitude adjustment is through prayer. Prayer can clarify issues, provide strength, and point you toward solutions. Prayer is a support group to end all support groups. It is always there, it can be used in any situation, it doesn't require expensive tools, and it works! Ask God for the attitude of gratitude. "May God, who gives this patience and encouragement, help you live in complete harmony with each other—each with the attitude of Christ Jesus toward the other. Then all of you can join together with one voice, giving praise and glory to God, the Father of our Lord Jesus Christ." (Rom. 15:5)

God knows your heart and wants you to follow the path to healing and joy. He can give you the strength. A patient once told me that God could show you how to make the "brain" change. But you need to ask, to seek, and, more importantly, to listen.

God answers prayer in many ways. It may be a booming bass voice from above, or it may be a whisper from a good friend. It may come as a magazine article that you just happen to pick up. It may come from a book you read. It may come as an afternoon talking with your mom about her midlife changes. It may come as an intuitive feeling. Use prayer to encourage day-to-day attitude adjustment.

"So then, since Christ suffered physical pain, you must arm yourselves with the same attitude he had, and be ready to suffer, too. For if you are willing to suffer for Christ, you have decided to stop sinning. And you won't spend the rest of your life chasing after evil desires, but you will be anxious to do the will of God."(1 Pet. 4:1–2)

Attitude Adjustment

What constitutes a "good" attitude toward menopause?
Knowing the following:

1. It is a normal, natural transition.
2. It is the end of reproduction, not of production.
3. Growing old is inevitable; growing up is optional.
4. I can choose; I have options.
5. I am not alone.
6. God has a plan for little old me.
7. A hot flash is a power surge.
8. I will not suffer from hardening of the attitude.
9. Research says successful traits include enthusiasm, passion, balance, focus, and togetherness.
10. Menopause is puberty with experience.

APTITUDE

The second A in the prescription for midlife success is Aptitude, the ability to gain knowledge and the willingness to learn what is going on in your body. The operative words here are ability and willingness. The limiting factor is usually not ability but willingness. No one cares more about your body than you do. You have to take time to learn how things function (even if on a superficial level), or you will have difficulty making smart decisions. Without a knowledge base about menopause, you are handicapped in dealing with it.

Not only is it important to learn the basics of your body functions, but it is also important to learn about your choices. If you are not aware of different treatment options, then you are at the mercy of those who present you with the choices. Daily, I hear patients say that their doctors never told them anything about alternatives to taking hormones. Time and time again, I have heard patients say that if they had known more about their choices they would have made vastly different decisions. No one will team these things for you. You have to make a concerted effort to acquire this knowledge.

I am preaching to the choir, because you wouldn't be reading this book if you weren't already interested in educating yourself. So I applaud you for that, but don't stop here. Read other books, and search the Internet. There are incredible resources available today, as opposed to ten years ago when it was as hard to find a book on menopause as it was to find a book on compassion in the IRS. Now the shelves are full of good references about every aspect of menopause.

Remember that she who learns only from herself has a fool for a teacher. Sixty-four percent of women can't name the hormones that play key roles in menopause, according to a 1998 Yankelovich poll of more than 1,000 women age forty and older, conducted for the University of Cincinnati. Forty-four percent say they don't know much about estrogen, and 65 percent say they have little knowledge about progesterone. These numbers are frightening! How can a woman make informed decisions about her health if she doesn't even know the basics? Educate yourself, go to seminars, read books, and talk to knowledgeable friends and family.

At the same time, be careful, because there is an overabundance of inaccurate, biased information floating around about menopause, especially on the Internet. View everything with a critical eye. Knowledge is not power, but the application of knowledge is power. Taking the knowledge and measuring it with a moral and ethical yardstick is wisdom. "The fear of the LORD is the beginning of knowledge. Only fools despise wisdom and discipline" (Prov. 1:7).

A newspaper once published this list (from an unknown author) of nine marks of an educated woman:

1. Has your education made you a friend of all good causes?
2. Has your education made you a brother to the weak?
3. Do you see anything to love in a little child?

4. Would a lost dog follow you in the street?
5. Do you enjoy being alone?
6. Do you believe in the dignity of labor?
7. Can you look into a mud puddle and see the blue sky?
8. Can you go out in the night, look up in the sky, and see beyond the stars?
9. Is your life linked with God?

Notice that nowhere does it ask about college degrees, professional organizations, or awards. Education is not about pieces of paper. It is about introspection, gathering facts, asking questions, making mistakes, assessing options, and following dreams. The biggest health care crisis in this country today is not AIDS, not cancer, and not heart disease. It is people not taking responsibility for making healthy lifestyle choices. The place to start is with education.

Action

The third component in the four A's is a call to Action. This has a double meaning. One is obvious; you have to do something to make something else happen. You have to take action. This is a simple concept, yet it is basic to success in dealing with the changes of menopause. You can't be a spectator and expect to glide through these changes. All of the information you glean is worthless unless you apply it. That is what I mean by action. You have to accumulate wisdom and knowledge and adapt it to your situation. Everyone is different, and what works for Aunt Geraldine may not work for you. That is why it is essential to take action. There is a huge gap between knowing what to do and doing it. Often that gap can become a chasm. It is easy to fall into the trap of inactivity, and there is no greater barrier to success.

The Epistle of James talks about faith without works. "Just as the body is dead without a spirit, so also faith is dead without good deeds"(James 2:26). Ideas, knowledge, and faith will die without action. Tony Robbins, a well-known motivational speaker, says, "If you always do what you have always done, then you will get what you have always gotten!"

If the task of "celebrating menopause" seems daunting, begin with baby steps. The hardest part of any chore is starting it. Begin today by taking the knowledge you have garnered from this book and apply just one of the principles. Next week adopt another; the following week, another. Soon you will be a veritable "Ms. Menopause," spreading the gospel of health and happiness to grouchy old folks worldwide! But you have to start. Edward Young said, "One of these days is none of these days."

Why do people fail to take action? One of the biggest reasons is fear of failure. What if it doesn't work? What if I find out something bad? What if I have to give up something I don't want to? For some it may actually be the fear of success! What if I change and my husband doesn't like it? What if I feel better and have nothing left to complain about? What is fear but False Expectations Appearing Real? In other words, the imagination is often much worse than the reality.

Don't let the fear of failure cause you to stagnate. That is the only true failure, the failure of inactivity. Every action begins with an idea, but that idea can die from inactivity. The two are intimately linked, and one cannot survive without the other. The most educated people in the world are impotent unless they apply their knowledge. What good is a guru who spends her entire day "thinking great thoughts"? She may be full of facts and philosophy but lacking in wisdom. Wisdom is taking knowledge and using it to make moral decisions, then acting on those decisions. It is not what we can do, it is what we *will* do that counts. The apostle James writes, "If you need wisdom-if you want to know what God wants ask him, and he will gladly tell you. He will not resent your asking." (James 1:5)

One of the most beautifully poetic treatises on wisdom is found in Psalm 119:96–106:

> Even perfection has its limits,
> but your commands have no limit.

Oh, how I love your law!
    I think about it all day long.
Your commands make me wiser than my enemies,
    for your commands are my constant guide.
Yes, I have more insight than my teachers,
    for I am always thinking of your decrees.
I am even wiser than my elders,
    for I have kept your commandments.
I have refused to walk on any path of evil,
    that I may remain obedient to your word.
I haven't turned away from your laws,
    for you have taught me well.
How sweet are your words to my taste;
    they are sweeter than honey.
Your commandments give me understanding;
    no wonder I hate every false way of life.
Your word is a lamp for my feet
    and a light for my path.
I've promised it once, and I'll promise again:
    I will obey your wonderful laws.

The Benefits of Action

David knew the power of action. While the whole army of Israel was immobilized, David went after that bad boy, Goliath. With God standing by him, he had no reason to procrastinate. He showed that inactivity could be fatal. The only way to make a difference was to accomplish the impossible. He did!

Jochebed, mother of Moses, didn't stand idly by as Pharaoh's army killed the male Jewish children. She took action, and a nation was led from captivity.

The five daughters of Zelophehad, whose story is told in Numbers, took action and petitioned Moses to grant them their father's inheritance, which would have otherwise been lost to them. Some jurists have declared it the oldest decided case "that is still cited as an authority."

Rahab, the harlot of Jericho, took action in hiding the spies of Israel because of her belief in their God, and for her actions she and her family were spared when the walls of Jericho came tumbling down.

Esther, Queen of the Persian Empire, took heroic action to prevent the massacre of her race.

Lydia, a successful businesswoman of Philippi, heard the message of Christ from Paul and didn't just embrace the idea; she took action and made her home the first meeting place for Christians in Europe.

Priscilla, a tentmaker with her husband, became one of the most influential women of the early Christian Church, not by her grand ideas or her scholarly theology, but by actively teaching her wisdom at Corinth and Ephesus.

These are biblical examples of numerous everyday women and men who took their passionate ideas and beliefs and transformed their lives and the lives of others through action.

James summarizes the importance of taking action in his epistle: "Dear brothers and sisters, what's the use of saying you have faith if you don't prove it by your actions? That kind of faith can't save anyone."(James 2:14)

The second part of the Action prescription involves moving-literally. The dreaded *E*-word. Exercise. God meant us to be mobile. You were designed to move. If you were meant to sit around all day, you would have been created as a spineless blob of protoplasm (although you might refer to your ex-husband this way). We should be physically active. This is such an important component of success in the menopause that I devote an entire chapter to exercise and its benefits.

Apothecary

The final A in my prescription for success in menopause is Apothecary. This stands for the many medicinals available to treat the symptoms of menopause. These include prescription medications, such as estrogen; natural products, such as black cohosh; and nutritional supplements, such as vitamin E. There is enough information on the subject to fill the next two chapters, so read on.

Action Challenge

Attitude: Tomorrow, jump out of bed. Instead of saying, "Good Lord, it's morning," shout, "*Good morning, Lord!*" It will start your day out right, and the look on your husband's face will be worth the effort!

Aptitude: Learn a new fun fact about your body to share with friends or loved ones. "Hey, Marge, did you know that if you took out my intestines and stretched them lengthwise they would go around this room three times?"

Action: Today walk around the room, tomorrow walk around the block, and the next day walk to the local health club and sign up.

Apothecary: Find something that looks and tastes like tree bark. Eat it. It is probably good for you and will keep you regular!

CHAPTER EIGHT

Treatment Options: Hormones

If you are reading this book, you are most likely doing so for one of two reasons. Either you are extremely bright and unbelievably discerning in your choice of reading material, or you are experiencing some symptom or symptoms of menopause or PMS that you wish to be rid of. In Chapter 2, I gave some options for PMS management. Now I want to do the same regarding menopause.

This chapter is a mini "how to" lesson on menopausal survival for those who do have bothersome symptoms. It is important to realize that not all will experience problems with menopause. There is no law that menopause is to be a trial by fire (or hot flash). However, for the 75 percent of women who have at least one bothersome symptom, this chapter is for you. Don't forget that this involves just one of the four A's, Apothecary. To achieve true balance and harmony, Attitude, Aptitude, and Action must be given equal attention. Review the prior chapters if that isn't clear.

The use of medications and/or herbs for the relief of menopausal problems is just a part of the solution. Proper nutrition, exercise, and state of mind all play an equal role in celebrating menopause.

The substances that will be discussed are an adjunct to other lifestyle choices. Medicines, herbs, and vitamins may work individually, but for a truly joyous time, all factors must be honored. Don't settle for surviving menopause; set a goal of rejoicing in menopause!

I am a recovering traditionalist. I was trained in a standard, structured curriculum as it pertained to menopause. My early training was based on the biomedical model of menopause, i.e., menopause is a hormone deficiency state. In the last several years I have adopted a life transition model for menopause, i.e., menopause is a normal, natural transition. This is reflected in my bias toward less invasive, complementary approaches to the problems of menopause. If it isn't broken don't fix it! But if it is broken, at least fix it in a way that doesn't make it worse!

Is One Treatment More Spiritual?

I use traditional hormone replacement in my practice a great deal. It is a proven, legitimate, and effective option for some women. Where my approach differs from some other practitioners is that I also offer and discuss proven, legitimate, nonhormonal alternatives for virtually every menopausal complaint. My role is to provide options and to make recommendations based on sound advice. I believe in the maxim, "First, do no harm."

Don't misunderstand my point. This complementary approach is my bias. I have not found anything in Scripture that disapproves or forbids the use of conventional drugs, hormones, or other modern medical triumphs. There is no moral superiority implied in my favoring "natural" treatments. A woman is no less spiritual if she uses HRT instead of herbs. I believe that God provides for all needs, and this may take several routes. I feel the admonition to treat the body as a temple must be considered when choosing what is right for you. My purpose is not to debate the theology of medical therapeutics. My purpose is to illuminate choices and allow a woman to use the discerning capacities granted to her by God to decide what is best for her.

In that context, I will first discuss traditional hormone replacement therapy and address when it is appropriate and when it is not. Then I will outline complementary approaches for a variety of specific symptoms. Part of my attraction to "natural" alternatives is the biblical example of using herbs and foods as medicines. Also, I am convinced that God has provided for our every need through the magnificence of creation.

There are some wonderful man-made medications available for a variety of ailments. God certainly works through men and women to provide these medications. God is great in supplying multitudes of choices and wonderfully effective options for menopausal complaints. Western cultures have become so enamored with technology and "pill" solutions that we have forgotten about the perfection of nature. The following pages are meant to stimulate you to explore and ask questions about what will be most effective for *you*.

Hormone Replacement Therapy

When I speak of hormone replacement therapy (HRT) I am talking about three hormones: estrogen, progesterone, and testosterone. The ovaries (and other tissues to a small degree) produce all three of these substances. HRT should be viewed as a medication. It is not a vitamin, cosmetic, or panacea. It is a prescription medication that should be used for specific reasons. It is ludicrous to suggest that every woman should be on HRT simply because she is menopausal. That is like saying all people should take blood pressure medicine just in case they develop hypertension. The first and most important questions to ask when investigating HRT are, what benefits can it offer, and conversely, what are the risks? As with any medication, the benefits have to outweigh the risks. There are some women who have certain problems that make HRT much too risky for any benefits (see Table 6 on the next page). All medications have side effects, and HRT is no exception.

There are women who realize substantial health gains from HRT. Just as all politics is local, so all medication use is individual. In other words, the use of HRT is a personal decision based on your

Table 6 Contraindication to Estrogen Use
Pregnancy
Breast Cancer
Uterine Cancer
Undiagnosed Vaginal Bleeding
Active Thrombphlebitis
Clotting Disorder
Acute Liver Disease
Chronic Liver Dysfunction

medical needs, past history, family history, and health philosophy. What is right for Aunt Marge may be very wrong for you!

There are basically two broad categories of legitimate reasons for using HRT. One is the short-term relief of symptoms. The second is the long-term health benefits, primarily osteoporosis prevention and the reduction of heart disease. If you are currently using HRT, or are considering using it, you must be able to identify which benefits exist for you. If you cannot, ask your health care worker or physician to pinpoint what benefits you are deriving from these drugs. If they cannot, either find a new doctor or get off the hormones! You must understand why you are taking these medications! If you don't, stop them until you get some answers.

There is no single substance available (including herbal and "natural" products) that, *by itself*, can control as many symptoms *and* provide as many prophylactic benefits as estrogen. Let's look at the types of estrogen available and the benefits and risks of each.

Estrogen in the body exists in primarily three forms: estrone (E1), estradiol (E2), and estriol (E3). The concentrations of each in the bloodstream vary at different times in a woman's life. There are probably about 20-25 different estrogens in a woman's body; however, most are in very small quantities and have very little effect. Estadiol is the predominant estrogen during the childbearing years, estrone predominates in the menopause, and estriol is increased during pregnancy.

In a wonderful book by Marcus Laux and Christine Conrad called *Natural Woman, Natural Menopause*, these estrogens are referred to as the "naturals." This is to separate them from the "synthetic" forms of estrogen, such as the ethinyl estradiol that is in many birth control pills. This distinction between natural and synthetic is an important one mainly because it is misunderstood. I explored this in the chapter on PMS, but it warrants repeating here, largely because of the debate raging among women over the merits of natural versus synthetic.

When you talk about hormones and someone says they are "natural," the first question you should ask is, "What do you mean by that?" There is tremendous confusion about what constitutes a natural substance. What you consider natural may be very different from what a manufacturer calls natural. There is no standard yet as to what that means. Anyone can label a product "natural," and no one regulates or controls what that means. It is the same phenomenon that occurred a few years back with "light." Foods were called "light," and it meant nothing until the government stepped in and legislated guidelines for labeling.

A simple definition I have found useful and accurate is that *natural* means it occurs in nature, as I explained in Chapter 2. An example is estradiol. It occurs naturally in a woman's body, but the actual substance that you take in a cream or pill form is made in the laboratory. It may have a plant as its origin, but in order for it to be utilized by the body, it has to be modified by a manufacturing process. It is indeed the same chemical substance that exists in the body, but it is not just plucked from the soil and ingested. This is in contrast to a substance like medroxyprogesterone acetate (Provera), which is a synthetic progestigen. Nowhere in nature can you find a naturally occurring molecule of medroxyprogesterone acetate. It is completely synthesized in the lab. Granted, it is broken down in your body and has progesterone-like action, yet the chemical itself is a man-made concoction. Many women today make decisions about the use of substances based on their labeling as "natural." Natural is good, but it may not always be what you think it is. Clarify in your own mind what constitutes "natural," and hold all substances to this standard.

Getting back to the estrogens. They are commonly used to treat symptoms or to provide long-term health benefits. Let's take a brief look at the ways in which they are utilized and further define the advantages and disadvantages.

When I am using the term *hormone replacement therapy* (HRT), I am referring to the use of both estrogen and progesterone. This combined use is essential for women who still have a uterus (and there are not many of you left!), because the use of estrogen alone increases the risk for cancer of the uterus. More on that later. In women who have had a hysterectomy it is OK to use estrogen by itself. However, even in these women the use of natural progesterone may have some benefits.

For years the controversy has raged on the pros and cons of using progestigens in women without a uterus. There are still those that think it is always a good idea to combine progestigens whenever estrogen is used; however, the bulk of the medical community feels that this is unnecessary and even potentially harmful. Many of the synthetic progestigens blunt the beneficial effect of estrogen on the heart. A large multicentered trial recently suggested that natural progesterone is much less likely to do this.

Immutable Rule 1: If you take estrogen and have a womb, take progesterone to avoid the tomb!

So, HRT may involve the use of estrogen by itself, estrogen plus progesterone, progesterone by itself, or testosterone plus any of the other regimens. Hormone replacement therapy or HRT technically refers to the use of both estrogen and a progestigen. When I use the term here it will mean just that. Estrogen replacement therapy (ERT) should apply to the use of estrogen alone. As stated, estrogen use by itself should be limited to those women who are minus their uterus. Not confusing at all, right! My bias is that HRT is a valid consideration for some women, but not necessarily the first or best choice. Virtually all the symptoms listed in chapter 4 can be addressed by traditional HRT.

Variety Is the Spice of Life

Estrogen can be given in several forms, preparations, and dosages. The most popular way of administering the drug is in pill form. Most people have heard of Premarin, the most-prescribed estrogen compound in pill form. This is the grandmother of estrogens and currently the most widely-used in the United States. It is a conjugated estrogen, meaning it is a mixture of many different chemical formulations of estrogens. It is derived from the urine of pregnant horses, and contains about 48 percent estrone (E1) and about 52 percent other estrogens native to the horse. The estrone (El) is converted in the body to estradiol (E2), which is the more potent form. Premarin comes in a variety of strengths (.3 mg, .625 mg, 1.25 mg, and 2.5 mg) and is now available in a single pill that combines it with a synthetic progestigen, called Prempro. I mention these brand names mainly because they are the most widely known, and many women think they are synonymous with HRT. They are not one and the same, however.

There are other options. Another pill is marketed under the trade name Estrace. It is different in that it is just estradiol (E2), identical to the E2 in a woman's body. It is micronized, or made into tiny particles, to allow it to be better absorbed from the stomach and intestines to the bloodstream. The only other "natural" estrogen pills are those containing E1, E2, and E3 (Tri-est) compounded by various pharmacies. I'll discuss those in a moment.

To bypass the gastrointestinal absorption route, a transdermal patch was developed that delivers estrogen directly to the bloodstream. This is a small adhesive patch about the size of a silver dollar that is worn on the skin and from which hormone is slowly released and absorbed through the skin. The advantage for some in using the patch is that it bypasses the stomach and intestines and is absorbed directly into the bloodstream. This avoidance of the "first pass effect" is important for people with gastrointestinal problems or who are taking multiple medications. There are several brand name patches available, and they all work in essentially the same way. One patch contains both estrogen and a progestigen and is now available in the United States. I have listed some of the currently marketed pills and their hormone makeup in Table 7.

TABLE 7
COMMON PRESCRIPTION ORAL ESTROGENS IN THE UNITED STATES

Name	Type of Estrogen.	Dose
*Premarin	conjugated estrogen	1mg, .625mg, 1.25mg, 2.5mg
+Estrace	estradiol (E2)	5mg, lmg, 2mg
+Estratab	esterified estrogens (mainly estrone)	.3mg,.625mg, 2.5mg
+Menest	esterified estrogens (mainly estrone)	.3mg,.625mg, 1.25mg, 2.5mg
+Orthoest	estropipate (estrone)	.75mg, 1.5mg
Combination tablets		
+Estratest	esterified estrogen	.625mg, 1.25mg
	methyltestosterone	1.25mg, 2.5mg
*Prempro/Premphase	conjugated estrogens	.625mg
	medroxyprogesteron acetate	2.5mg, 5mg
+Tri-est(cream or capsule)		
Micronized Estrone	estrone	
Micronized Estradiol	estradiol	1.5mg to 5mg total estrogen
Micronized Estriol	estriol	

+plant derived
*contains horse estrogens

Source: 1999 Physician's Desk Reference

I want to point out a couple of pills that do have unique characteristics. One pill is a combination of both estrogen and testosterone. Testosterone, commonly thought of as the male hormone, is produced by the ovary and is responsible for a variety of effects. The most relevant effects for the menopausal woman are enhancement of libido and a sense of wellbeing. It should be noted that the testosterone in these pills is a synthetic concoction called methyltestosterone, which differs from the "natural" testosterone in several creams.

Another unique pill is the combination pill of Premarin and Provera, called Prempro. This was created basically for two reasons: (1) to make taking HRT easier, and (2) to attempt to circumvent one of the most bothersome side effects of HRT, the resumption of periods. The most common combined regimen for using estrogen and progestigen is to take the estrogen every day and the progesterone 10-14 days out of the month. On this regimen the vast majority of women will continue having periods for as long as they are taking the hormones. This means you could be ninety-two years old and running to the grocery store at midnight for an emergency maxi-pad purchase. This is not something most ninety-two year olds want to do with their evenings!

A wise person then came up with the idea (I don't know for sure, but I bet it was a woman) of using the estrogen and progesterone on a daily basis to still get the benefits, but hopefully eliminate the bleeding. And it worked . . . some of the time . . . for some of the women. So this combination pill was developed and has definitely had an impact on prescribing habits. The twin sister of Prempro is Premphase. This combination pill is the same dosing schedule of traditional HRT, and most women will have withdrawal bleeds on this. Note that Estrace, Orthoest, and Estratab are plant-derived estrogens.

Don't forget the rule: If you have a uterus and are taking estrogen, then you must be on some form of progestigen also (preferably the natural progesterone). If you don't have a uterus, estrogen alone or progesterone alone are options.

Injections and Implants

Another mode of delivering estrogen, progesterone, and testosterone is through injections. This is a popular method among women who have had a hysterectomy, but should not be used by those who have been able to hold on to their uterus. The uterine bleeding with this method is unpredictable, and the effect on the uterine lining is not well documented. Using injectable hormones when a uterus is in place is risky business. However, in those women who have had a hysterectomy, it can be a viable option.

The injections are administered on a monthly schedule and consist of many different dosages and combinations. The medications are in a medium that allows for its slow release over three to four weeks. Many women like the injections for the freedom of not having to take something every day. Also the injections are helpful in women who can't take medicines by mouth or are on multiple medications that may interfere with the absorption of oral tablets. Injections go straight into the bloodstream and don't have the beneficial effect on blood lipids that the oral hormones do.

They are very effective in treating symptoms, and if used consistently, can help prevent osteoporosis. The biggest drawback to the injections is that some women experience a higher dose release initially (a rush of medicine) and then it tapers off quickly. This creates a roller coaster effect for the hormones in the bloodstream and is reflected at times in a seesaw battle of emotions. Most estrogens used in injections are synthetic and carry the known risks of estrogen use.

Although not approved by the FDA for this purpose, subdermal implants of estrogen and testosterone are available from compounding pharmacies and widely used, especially in certain, parts of the country. They are slid under the skin in a two-minute office procedure utilizing topical anesthesia. It is important to note that the FDA has approved the specific drugs for use, however, just not in this particular delivery system. It's like using Skin-So-Soft as a mosquito repellent. It works well in this capacity, yet that is not what it was designed for. Simply stated, the pellets contain the same estrogen and testosterone, just packaged differently. Again, in my opinion, these pellets should not be used in women who have all their parts (uterus). The long-term effect on the endometrium (lining of the uterus) is not known and the bleeding pattern is unpredictable. Many of the pellets are designed to release their hormones over a four-to-six-month period as they dissolve. Studies from Europe have shown consistent and reliable blood levels of hormones from the pellet implants. They are convenient, effective, and expensive.

Tri-est

Another method of administration of estrogen that is gaining in popularity is creams, in particular, the Tri-est cream. Jonathan Wright, MR, originated the Tri-est formulation about fifteen years ago. It is composed of a mixture of estrone (El), estradiol (E2), and estriol (E3), the same estrogens that predominate in a woman's system. The mixture is compounded by a pharmacist in a ratio of eight parts E3 to one part E2 and one part E1. The theory behind this mixture is that the E3 supposedly protects against some of the harmful effects of the other estrogens. Theoretically, this would make the preparation effective, with fewer side effects, and decreased potential for danger. There is some evidence that estriol may have less of a negative effect on the risk for breast cancer than estradiol; however, there have been no large well-done studies in women that absolutely confirm that estriol (E3) has this ability.

It is important to make the distinction between a lower risk of causing a problem and an actual protective effect. There is some data that suggests an association between high levels of E3 and the remission of breast cancer, yet this is far from conclusive. It is a gross distortion to say the present information supports the idea that E3 protects against breast cancer. The information is observational (much being from animal studies), and the relationship between E3 and breast cancer is far from definitive. It is one thing to provide data that shows an association between two events, and quite another to show a true cause-and-effect relationship. It can be said, however, that it appears that E3 is at least less likely to cause side effects than its cousins E2 and E1. Can Tri-est *cream* prevent osteoporosis? There are no large reliable studies that answer yes to that question. Tri-est requires a prescription and only certain pharmacies are willing and able to make this preparation.

Bio-identical Plant Estrogens

Estrone, estriol, and estradiol are available as oral, bioidentical, plant-derived products. They require a prescription and have to be made by a compounding pharmacy. Dr. Joel Hargrove of Vanderbilt University has published several studies showing the effectiveness of these formulations in treating symptoms of menopause. The advantage is that they are equivalent to the body's estrogen. They are converted from plant sources in the lab, but the final product packaged in capsules is "bio-identical" to a woman's own estrogen. For example, Tri-est *capsules* are available from compounding pharmacies. The bio-availability and absorption of this preparation is somewhat different than the cream, and some women prefer a tablet instead of the cream.

Many women choose to use these compounds, as they are natural in the sense that they are equivalent to the body's estrogen. The Tri-est formulation, with the predominant estrogen being E3, is not magical in its effects. Like any estrogen use, it has benefits and risks. In reality the majority of the benefits from Tri-est originate from the E2 (estradiol) content. This is the most biologically active form of the hormone. Any protective effect from the E3 (estriol) is still theoretical.

Cream Wars

Another unanswered question fueling controversy in the hormone wars is, do the creams get into the bloodstream enough to have a beneficial effect on symptoms and bones?

Advocates of the creams cite studies that evaluate both blood and salivary estrogen levels and say, "Yes, there is evidence that adequate levels are achieved." And their data supports that. Opponents of cream use state that there are multiple studies that show very little of the hormones actually get into the bloodstream. And their data supports that. (Can't we all just get along?) My guess is that the tremendous variation in these results is largely due to different testing methods, different cream formulations, and the individual variations in women's physiology.

All facets of these studies should be analyzed. For example, some studies may only have a handful of subjects while others gather data from a larger sample. Patients beware: Assessing all of these factors can be complicated. Studies are ongoing about the validity of cream use. For now, we can say that definite symptomatic relief (hot flashes, mood changes, etc.) can be obtained by some with the use of the creams. There is presently no convincing data on the ability of estrogen and progesterone creams to prevent osteoporosis and heart disease. Again I refer back to one of my original themes: God has provided a multitude of options for women, so don't use a cookie cutter approach. Educate yourself about options, and then experiment and see what works best for you.

Which is the best approach to HRT? Well, there is no best approach. The best way is what works for you and provides the health benefits you require. In addition to the overall estrogenic effects they all share, each method has its advantages and disadvantages. Whether it is a pill, patch, pellet, or cream, the choice is yours.

There are a variety of ways of evaluating its effectiveness once you have made the decision to use HRT. The best way is how you feel! Use your internal gauge to assess if it is right for you. I place a tremendous amount of importance on a woman's perception, intuition, and feelings. Often these intuitive feelings are much more valuable than numbers from a blood test. Granted some tests are valuable in assessing certain parameters, but I would much rather know how a woman is feeling about her HRT than know her estradiol level.

So, estrogen can be swallowed, shot in the rear end, implanted in your tum-tum, or stuck on your *derriere*. And it comes in a variety of flavors and combinations. There are undeniable benefits to using estrogens. They are very effective in eliminating symptoms, decreasing bone loss and the incidence of fractures, and lowering cholesterol and the propensity for heart disease. These benefits are well-documented in many scientific studies, and those who question these particular effects haven't studied the issue and are handcuffed by their own prejudices. Also, there is some evidence that

HRT *may* have a preventive effect on colon cancer, and *may* be beneficial in slowing down or even preventing Alzheimer's disease. These findings are preliminary and certainly can't be taken as the gospel truth, but it will be interesting to follow these developments.

There is a tremendous amount of money and effort being thrown into hormone research, and it is estimated that the next few years may produce twenty to thirty new hormone preparations. In addition, it is hoped that many of the risks of estrogen will be accurately elucidated over the next decade. For women considering some form of treatment now, the best advice I can give is to consider options, evaluate benefits and risks, and consult with a trusted, knowledgeable, and caring health care worker.

The Down Side

Every party has a pooper, and every drug has a down side. No medication is without side effects, and estrogen, be it El, E2, E3, or conjugated estrogens, is no exception. The specter of cancer pervades any discussion of HRT. In a recent survey, fear of cancer was the second leading cause both of not taking hormones and of stopping them once they are started. A recent Gallup poll of middle-aged women showed that close to 40 percent thought they would eventually die from breast cancer. The reality is that only 4 percent will! This fear of breast cancer has become so pervasive in our society that some women are demanding prophylactic mastectomies to remove their chance of ever battling the evil.

The scientific community agrees that the use of estrogen alone increases the risk for cancer of the *uterus*. The debate rages on about the influence of estrogen and breast cancer.

Breast Cancer

The different camps on either side of the breast cancer issue are entrenched and passionate. The reason that the general public is confused is because doctors are confused. Does the use of estrogen

TABLE 8
KNOWN RISK FACTORS FOR BREAST CANCER

Family history (mother or sister)
Early puberty
Late menopause
Delayed childbearing (first child after age 35)
No pregnancies
Age over 60
Prior breast cancer

Potential Risk Factors (under investigation)
Obesity
High fat diet
Alcohol use
ERT

promote breast cancer? Is the risk dependent on the type and duration of estrogen use? Can the studies that look at the effect of birth control pills on breast cancer be applied to ERT?

Let me state assuredly that the answer to all these questions is a resounding . . . we don't know! How's that for clarity?

The good news is there are a couple of large, ongoing studies that will finally give some hard answers to this difficult question. The bad news is we probably won't have any meaningful data from these for ten or more years.

To illustrate the dilemma, look at a few of the larger previous studies and their conclusions. A composite reanalysis of data from fifty-one studies representing 90 percent of the world literature on the relationship between estrogen use and breast cancer published in the British medical journal, *The Lancet*, had these conclusions: The annual breast cancer risk increased by 2.8 percent for each year of delayed menopause (>53), and the annual breast cancer risk increased by 2.3 percent for each year of ERT use. The breast cancer risk after five or more years of ERT use was increased by 35 percent. After stopping ERT five or more years are required to return to never-user risk.[1]

A series of papers in which data from many different studies was pooled to make conclusions (called a meta analysis) shows again the inconsistency in the conclusions. Armstrong (1988) showed no effect of ERT on breast cancer.[2] A study by Dupont and Page (1991) gave a resounding "maybe."[3] Steinberg (1991) showed a 30 percent increase in the incidence of breast cancer after a fifteen-year use of ERT,[4] and Colditz (1993) assessed a "slight" increase after ten years of use.[5]

Case controlled studies, including the CASH study, Stanford in 1995, Kaufman in 1991, and Palmer in 1991, all concluded that there was no increased risk of breast cancer in postmenopausal estrogen users.[6]

So what do you do? It is obvious that there are still no clear answers. Many prominent scientists believe estrogen use has absolutely contributed to the rise in breast cancer. A similar number of people feel just the opposite. Understand your choices. All this data and all these numbers mean little to the woman trying to define what is best for her long-term health. If you are afraid of ERT whether it is justified fear or not, my experience is that your compliance on an ERT regimen will be poor. Therefore if you have a great concern about ERT specifically as it relates to breast cancer, educate yourself about other options. It is not an all-or-nothing decision. You do have choices. With respect to breast cancer, it is extremely important to keep the risks in a proper perspective.

What can be said then? Almost all of the studies agree that the short-term use of HRT (five years or less) provides no additional risk for developing breast cancer.

The contributors to breast cancer risk are multifactorial. In other words, there are many factors that must be considered when determining your individual risk. Some doctors consider estrogen's role like a fertilizer. It doesn't initiate a breast cancer, but if a cancer starts, estrogen may accelerate its growth.

Table 8 lists some of the common risk factors for breast cancer. Risk factors can be deceptive in that they may lull you into a false sense of security. If you don't have any of these known risk factors, you cannot be complacent. Seventy percent of women who develop breast cancer have no identifiable risk factor! Eighty percent of women diagnosed with breast cancer have no family history of the disease!

Know Your Risk

Your individual risk is a mix between your genetic make-up (family history) and the environment (foods you eat, medicines you take, and things you are exposed to). While you can't change your genes, you can alter other risk factors. Many believe these factors are more important than genetics in determining your risk.

Few breast cancers are caused solely by genetic changes. Genetics are much more important for determining the propensity for cancer to arise when certain environmental conditions are present. This is comparable to all the conditions being in place for the formation of a tornado, including wind, temperature, and pressure changes. That propensity exists often, yet only when they combine in a certain fashion does a tornado actually form. So it is with breast cancer. The genetics provide the conditions, and the environment (what we eat, medicines we take, chemicals we work around, etc.) determines whether a cancer will form. There are many other factors that play a role, such as the immune system. But breast cancer is usually not caused by one single element.

Dr. Graham Colditz, author of one of the studies previously cited and associate professor of medicine at Harvard Medical School, effectively puts risk into terms that are easily understood: "Approximately one additional woman in one thousand per year will get breast cancer while on estrogen compared to women who are not on hormones."[7]

If this level of risk is unacceptable for you, look to the many other choices available.

Cautions

I have already mentioned that women who have a uterus should rarely, if ever, use estrogen by itself because of the known risk of cancer of the uterus. When estrogen is coupled with the proper dosage and duration of a progestigen, this risk becomes the same as that of the general population. There is no credible evidence that the use of HRT increases a woman's risk for cancer of the cervix or cancer of the ovary. It is established that the use of HRT can make a woman more susceptible to gall bladder disease. Women who have a tendency to form blood clots should not use HRT. The hormones are broken down and metabolized by the liver, so if a woman has any active liver disease such as hepatitis, she should never use HRT.

PROGESTERONE

The second major hormone that is important to include in the discussion of HRT is progesterone. Progesterone is the "counterbalancing" hormone in the normal menstrual cycle. I have already mentioned this several times; however, it is important for you to understand some differences in terminology. Progesterone is a specific chemical that has specific effects in the body. Table 9 lists many of the known actions of progesterone.

A progest*igen* refers to any substance that has progesterone-like action. It is a generic term for many different drugs, including synthetics like medroxyprogesterone acetate and norethindrone. These are progestigens that are commonly used in birth control pills and/or HRT. They were developed largely to facilitate their oral absorp-

TABLE 9
ACTIONS OF PROGESTERONE

Provides suitable environment for the nourishment of the developing embryo
Acts as an anti-estrogen on the uterus
Decreases estrogen receptors in the uterus
Binds to androgen receptors
Serves as a building block for other hormones
Blocks estrogen stimulation of breast epithelial cells
Increase HDL cholesterol
Decrease LDL cholesterol

tion so that they could be effectively given in pill form. Progesterone is poorly absorbed in the digestive tract. If its chemical structure is slightly altered, it becomes more bio-available and also, because it is now a "new" drug, able to be patented.

However, by altering the structure you also change its effects on the body. Synthetic progestigens have many of the same actions that are seen with "natural" progesterone; however, the synthetic progestigens have a plethora of adverse reactions that make their use less than ideal for a lot of women. Bloating, depression, breast tenderness, abdominal cramping, and mood changes all have been associated with synthetic progestigens.

If you must take a progestigen because you are taking estrogen, then the pure progesterone, now available in a tablet form, is your best option. The cream has actually been around for about fifty years and is manufactured in the lab from soybeans or yam. It is the same chemical as progesterone in your body except it is manufactured in the lab. The soybean or yam extract contains a chemical called diosgenin, which is converted to the progesterone by a series of chemical reactions. You cannot do this in your body because you lack the proper enzymes to convert diosgenin to progesterone. In other words, don't buy an over-the-counter product that contains only Mexican yam extract or diosgenin because your body cannot convert this to progesterone. You are getting a good moisturizer, and that is about it. The best thing to do when you go shopping for a true progesterone cream is to look on the package for a list of the ingredients. If it doesn't specifically say, "contains progesterone," stay away from it.

Crinone, a natural progesterone gel, is a prescription drug that is administered vaginally. In England this preparation is used in cyclic hormone replacement therapy and is beginning to be used on a daily basis to counterbalance estrogen. In the United States, Crinone progesterone gel is approved for use in cases of amenorrhea, or lack of periods. There are no studies on the effectiveness of Crinone gel in relieving any symptoms of menopause.

Some people propose that the majority of menopausal symptoms are a result of estrogen dominance or progesterone deficiency. These same folks promote progesterone cream with an almost religious fervor as a cure for whatever ails you. At times these pronouncements sound much like the "medicine show" salesmen of the Old West. There is no doubt that natural progesterone cream has a place in the treatment of perimenopausal and menopausal symptoms; however, I am skeptical of the purported breadth of the "miraculous" cures.

A recent paper presented at the annual meeting of the American Society of Reproductive Medicine showed progesterone cream to be more effective than placebo in eliminating hot flashes. This is one of the few good studies examining the cream and its use in menopause. There are many individual testimonials and anecdotal reports of effectiveness. When you search the world literature for studies on progesterone cream you find a paucity of good scientific work that shows the benefit of the cream over a placebo. Even the proponents of natural progesterone cream cite references to support their claims that refer to natural progesterone, but in the micronized pill form. Because these are different delivery systems, it is improper to compare the results obtained with one to the other.

In my practice, natural progesterone cream is most useful in the treatment of hot flashes and breast tenderness. I have also used it with some success in PMS. These are individual reports, and I certainly can't back them up with formal scientific studies. Even the European literature, which is commonly ahead of America in alternative approaches, is remarkably sparse in clinical studies on the cream. Studies are presently being conducted to properly assess the benefits of cream.

One area to be cautious about is the supposed relationship between natural progesterone cream and osteoporosis. Some authors, notably Dr. John Lee, state that natural progesterone cream can not only prevent osteoporosis, but may even rebuild lost bone. He is the only one to report actual clinical data to support these conclusions, and that data is questionable. Progesterone does bind to receptors in the bone, but that is a long way from saying it builds bone! A paper that showed the positive influence of cream on hot flashes also stated that in their sample there was no effect on bone loss from the cream over the year that the patients were followed. To date there is no credible evidence that states progesterone *cream* is effective in preventing osteoporosis.

Understand the distinction here. Progesterone, the chemical in your body, can affect bone and may help thwart bone loss in the menopause. The debate is whether the *cream* form of progesterone gets into your bloodstream and to the bone in a high enough concentration to actually mimic this effect. The current data would suggest it doesn't. I caution patients not to rely on this as their sole protection against this potentially horrible disease. Studies are currently underway in several centers to try to validate Dr. Lee's claims, especially in the area of osteoporosis prevention. There may be some additive benefit of oral natural progesterone on bone, but only time will tell.

The Benefits

Natural progesterone capsules are useful in several situations. First, pure progesterone has few of the side effects of synthetic products. It can be used instead of medroxyprogesterone acetate (Provera) to provide all of the protective benefits. With the advent of the micronized progesterone tablet, options for women have been expanded. Many who cannot tolerate synthetics do very well on the natural. A large study showed the micronized progesterone had a more favorable effect on lowering cholesterol than synthetic progestins, and protected the uterus adequately.[9] In those taking progesterone, the use of the natural progesterone oral capsule only makes sense.

Some have advocated the use of progesterone alone for the treatment of menopausal symptoms. I agree that it is helpful in some women with hot flashes and breast tenderness. I have several patients who use the cream exclusively for these reasons and are doing quite well. So, it has its place. It is not a panacea, but it can be helpful in certain women in certain situations. Specifics on dosages will be given later.

Pump You Up

Testosterone is traditionally identified as the male hormone, because it is produced in much higher quantities in men. When

Table 10
Currently Available Prescription Progestins

Brand name	Contents	Dosage
Amen	medroxyprogesterone acetate	10mg
Aygestin	norethindrone acetate	5mg
Cycrin	medroxyprogesterone acetate	2.5mg, 5mg, 10mg
Crinone gel	micronized progesterone	4 %, 8%
Depo-provera (injectable)	medroxyprogesterone acetate	various
Micronor (birth control)	norethindrone	.35mg
Prometrium	micronized progesterone	100mg, 200mg
Provera	medroxyprogesterone acetate	2.5mg, 5mg, 10mg

Nonprescription Progesterone Creams*

Brand name	Manufacturer	Location
Pro-Gest	Professional &Technical Service	Portland, Ore.
Angel care	Angel Care, USA	Atlanta, Ga.
Probalance	Springboard	Monterray, Calif
Natural Balance	South Market Services	Atlanta, Ga.
Equillibrium	Equillibrium Lab	Boca Raton, Fla.
Edenn	SNM	Norcross, Ga.
Phytogest	Karuna Corp.	Novato, Calif.
Serenity	Health and Science	Crewfordvil, Fla.
Restored Balance	Thymates, Inc	Atlanta, Ga.

*not a complete list. All products listed have 400-500mg/oz. Progesterone determined by Aeron Lifecycles Lab.

you hear of athletes using performance-enhancing drugs, this usually refers to a high dose of a form of testosterone. However, the ovary, that powerhouse of production, makes testosterone also. The adrenal glands, which sit on top of both kidneys, also produce testosterone and its precursors. So, the female body does have testosterone flowing in its veins. Some women actually produce an excess of testosterone and suffer from its effects: acne, oily skin, hair growth (where you don't want it), enlargement of the clitoris, and even deepening of the voice.

Testosterone has long been associated with a sense of well-being and libido when it is produced in balance with the other hormones. Testosterone continues to be produced after menopause; however, the amounts can vary. Testosterone production falls dramatically in women who have had their ovaries removed. Because of this dramatic drop of testosterone, these women are more likely to suffer from decreased sex drive than someone who retains their functioning ovaries. Libido is a complex drive with many contributing factors. Hormones actually play a relatively minor role. (My extensive research has shown that the number one cause of a decreased libido is . . . husbands!) However, there is a legitimate place for replacing testosterone when it is low.

How do you know if it is low? The best test is the measurement of free or active testosterone in saliva. Serum tests for testosterone and its precursors are helpful but mainly show the bound or inactive hormone. Assessing testosterone levels can help clarify whether this is a significant player in libido problems. If a woman is symptomatic and her levels are low, then it is appropriate to consider testosterone replacement.

There are currently four common ways of administering testosterone. They mimic the methods of administering estrogen: pills, pellets, shots, and creams. My bias is using the pure testosterone creams because you can use a lower dose and change it with fewer side effects. I use a 2 percent testosterone cream compounded by the pharmacy, with approximately a half teaspoon rubbed on the abdomen or buttocks once or twice a day. Levels can be monitored by saliva testing, but again I rely largely on what the woman is experiencing and feeling in addition to the numbers.

There are multiple studies that show the benefits of androgen replacement, but there are potential side effects. If an excess of testosterone exists you may suffer from the signs already mentioned: acne, oily skin, weight gain, hair growth. There is also evidence that rising levels of testosterone may increase triglycerides and alter liver function. Very high dosages of testosterone are what the muscle-bound bodybuilders use, and the dangers from this are legion. The dosages used for hormone replacement in women are vastly lower than those used by the Hulk wannabes, so they won't turn women into Arnold Schwarzenegger look-alikes.

Action Challenge

Answer this question: Why would I consider taking a medicine for menopause? Is it for symptom relief or long-term health benefits (or both)?

CHAPTER NINE

Treatment Options: Alternative Approaches

If you are hoping to find a discussion, of crystals, chants, and other wacko alternative medicine mumbo jumbo, you'd best look elsewhere. I gravitate toward the term *complementary approaches* because this describes more accurately the nonexclusivity of these regimens. It is not an either/or decision. You can use HRT and herbs and vitamins together, or you can use herbs and vitamins exclusively. Life is about choices, and this book is about choices.

Immutable Rule 2: Women rejoice; you have a choice!

Certainly you have the option to do nothing (and for some that is a legitimate choice), but, more importantly, you have the ability (and soon the knowledge) to look at all the fabulous foods, herbs, and vitamins that God has provided and utilize them to maximize your health.

Listen to the advice of Solomon in Proverbs 3:7–8: "Don't be impressed with your own wisdom. Instead, fear the LORD and turn your back on evil. Then you will gain renewed health and vitality." He doesn't condemn the use of your wisdom; just don't get a big head about it. Also, Solomon notes, for the best advice and guidance, listen to the Lord and avoid those who say wrong. That is sound advice for menopause and life in general.

Biblical Guidance

Does the Bible say anything about herbs and foods as medicines? You bet it does! In Revelation 22:2, John writes about the river "coursing down. the center of the main street. On each side of the river grew a tree of life, bearing twelve crops of fruit, with a fresh crop each month. The leaves were used for medicine to heal the nations." Symbolic, yes, but the meaning is not lost on its practical application. The Old Testament is full of examples, as in this passage from 2 Kings 20:7, "Then Isaiah said to Hezekiah's servants, `Make an ointment from figs and spread it over the boil.' They did this, and Hezekiah recovered!" Jeremiah 8:22 talks about a "balm" (herbal treatment) as a symbol for spiritual healing. "Is there no balm in Gilead? Is there no physician there? Why is there no healing for the wounds of my people?"

In specifically applying natural medicines to menopause, it is helpful to list the different herbs and foodstuffs by the symptoms they address. I will examine many of the common symptoms and present complementary approaches to those specific symptoms. There is overlap, as one herb or vitamin may be useful for several symptoms. Also, and very importantly, I have included only treatments that I have found successful and that have documented scientific validation.

This is by no means a comprehensive list of all possible natural or herbal treatments for symptoms, but it is bound by the maxim of scientifically-proven effectiveness. The biggest problem women face in choosing complementary therapies is separating the wheat from the chaff. What works, and what doesn't? I have carefully surveyed the current literature and assembled only those remedies that are scientifically proven to be valid. Not all herbal approaches are legitimate, or maybe it is better to say that many of the claims regarding herbal potency are invalid. Herbs and plants are all part of

God's great master plan. For us the key is how to utilize them safely and appropriately.

PHYTOESTROGENS

There is a category of foods that have such a broad positive effect on menopausal problems that they form the foundation of any natural program. These are the foods that contain phytoestrogens. Phytoestrogens are plant substances that abound in soy products, legumes, flaxseed, whole grains, beans, vegetables, and some fruits. The two main types of phytoestrogens that we are concerned with are lignans and isoflavones. Phytoestrogens are weak estrogens; however, their ability to express biological activity in the body is the same as estrogens produced by the body.[1]

A study published in the journal *Obstetrics and Gynecology* in 1998 showed that after twelve weeks of ingesting 60 g a day of soy products, 44 percent of 104 women experienced the elimination of their hot flashes.[2] Messina in 1991 showed that a cup of soybeans a day could increase the vaginal cell maturation,[3] which is an indication of the estrogen effect on the cells lining the vagina. This is

TABLE 11
PHYTOESTROGEN CONTENT OF COMMON SOY PRODUCTS

Food	Isoflavone content (mcg/g)
Tofu	232
Soy sauce	13
Soy milk	44
Soybean sprouts	368
Soybean, green	1285
Soybean paste	330
Miso paste	642
Soy hot dog	188

Adapted from K. Reinli and G. Block, "Phytoestrogen content of foods—a copendium of literature values," *Nutr Cancer* 26 (1996): 123–48.

important in resolving vaginal dryness and pain during intercourse. Anderson and colleagues showed, in 1995, that a diet rich in soy (phytoestrogens) could lower total cholesterol, LDL cholesterol (the bad guys) and triglycerides.[4] Aldercreutz, in an article published in the Annuls of Medicine, provided data that suggested that isoflavones and lignans could reduce the incidence of breast, colon, and prostate cancers.[5]

The effect of phytoestrogens on bone has not been well-studied. There is some cross-cultural data looking at the lower incidence of osteoporosis in cultures that consume a great deal of soy and soy products; however, cause and effect cannot be stated with confidence. There is no evidence that an increase in phytoestrogen consumption will increase your risk of uterine or breast cancer.

What is the practical application of all this data? Table 11 lists the phytoestrogen content of some common soy foods. The evidence is compelling that women who suffer from hot flashes and vaginal dryness should first increase their dietary intake of these products before looking at other solutions. They may not need to look any further! If you hate tofu and soy, try various legumes, chickpeas, or whole grains. (See Table 12.)

Flaxseed oil is available as a supplement and is a good source of lignans. The best way to utilize flaxseed oil is to add it directly to foods. It shouldn't be used as cooking oil as it is easily broken down in the heat. A great way to use the flaxseed oil is to substitute it for other oils in making salad dressing. Flaxseed oil is also the richest supplier of omega 3 fatty acids, known to have a protective effect on the heart. Most studies report that a tablespoon of the oil a day provides you with the amount of phytoestrogens needed to combat hot flashes. The amount that works for you may vary, and, as with all these remedies, don't expect overnight success.

Another option is direct supplimentation with isoflavone containing tablets. Promensil is a proprietary product that contains 40 mg isoflavones, which is an amount shown to be effective in several studies. Most research shows the benefits after four or more weeks of use.

Start here. It is simple to do and effective. Tablets that contain concentrated isoflavones can supplement a diet low in these substances. This is a convenient way to increase the consumption of these helpful chemicals without loading up on other foods.

Next, let's look at common individual symptoms of menopause and their effective, scientifically valid, and safe treatments.

TABLE 12
COMMON PHYTOESTROGEN CONTAINING FOODS

Soybeans and soy products	Cereal bran
Tofu	Whole cereals
Whole grains	Clover sprouts
Chickpeas	Beans
Legumes	Tempeh
Flaxseed	

HOT FLASHES

Hot flashes, surges of energy, heat waves, prickly heat—a rose by any other name is still a rose. The hot flash is the single most common symptom of the menopause. It is estimated that up to 75 percent of women experience this phenomenon to some degree (pun intended). A vital distinction is understanding what a hot flash is and what it isn't. Many women are confused by what constitutes a true hormonal hot flash. Typically it begins suddenly in the upper chest and gallops headward, spreading its warmth and joy. Sweating and a perceptible increase in skin temperature often accompany it. It may occur once a day, or it may occur a hundred times a day. It is not the continual feeling of warmth that many women describe. Every day I have women report that they are just generally warmer than their husbands or colleagues, but this is more a steady state metabolic variation than the explosive flashing characterized by a hormonal hot flash.

The question I get asked often is, "When do you do something about the hot flashes?"

The answer is, "Whenever they bother you!" No one ever died from hot flashes, although many have wished they would. It is confusing to women who don't have a problem with these to understand the difficulty that hot flashes may cause.

Alice, a top executive with a local bank, relayed her first experience with a hot flash. She was making a presentation to the bank's board of directors, and at an important sequence in the presentation, she suddenly felt that her head was on fire. She felt her 24-hour antiperspirant was on its third day! She fought the urge to rip her clothes off, which no doubt would have made an impression on the board, and pressed forward. Not only was she spooked by not knowing what was going on, she had never before "let them see her sweat." She was a control fanatic, which was why she had risen in the bank hierarchy so fast. But now, for the first time, she felt out of control. She was able to laugh about it when she came and saw me, but only after I reassured her that she could control and possibly eliminate the flashes forever. Here are the options I presented.

Vitamin E

Vitamin E has long been used to eliminate hot flashes. As far back as 1949, studies showed the effectiveness of vitamin E for hot flashes and other menopausal symptoms.[6] The exact mechanism of how it works is unknown, but I have successfully used it in my practice for years. Most of the scientific data suggest a minimum dosage of 800 units of D-alpha tocopherol daily is effective. If most of the hot flashes occur at night, as they commonly do, take the vitamin E as a single dose at bedtime. Vitamin E is somewhat better absorbed if taken with food, even better if there is a little fat in the food. Now isn't it great to have something good to say about fat! Vitamin E is a fat-soluble vitamin meaning it has the potential to be stored in the body in fat cells; however, dosages of up to 2,000 IU a day have been shown to be safe. Dietarily, vitamin E can be found in vegetable oils, almonds, walnuts, margarine, spinach, lettuce, and onions.

Vitamin E is also associated with a variety of other health benefits. It is a powerful antioxidant and has been shown to decrease the incidence of heart disease in certain individuals. It may protect from some types of cancers. Most women who successfully eliminate their hot flashes with vitamin E could care less about the heart protective benefits; they are just glad to be cooler!

Black Cohosh

Cimicifuga Racemosa, or black cohosh, is one of the most studied and utilized herbs for the elimination of hot flashes. Black cohosh is a beautiful, long, drooping raceme with delicate white flowers, and is native to the United States. The medicinal part of the plant is the dried root.

I am a fan of a product called Remifemin, which is a proprietary product that contains a standardized dose of triterpenes, the active ingredient of black cohosh. This particular product has been widely used in Germany for years and has valid studies that support its effectiveness and safety. A recent article in the *Journal of Women's Health* concludes that Cimicifuga Racemosa is extremely effective in treating hot flashes and other menopausal symptoms.[7]

Several randomized, double blind, placebo-controlled studies have demonstrated the effectiveness of Remifemin on hot flashes, vaginal dryness, and mood changes.[8] One of the most interesting and telling studies was published in 1988. It compared Remifemin with estriol (E3) and Premarin, and tested their effects on controlling various menopausal symptoms. This study used the Kupperman Menopausal Scale, a long-validated measure of symptom intensity. The results showed that there was no significant difference among any of the treat-ment groups, and *all* were effective in reducing the frequency and in-tensity of symptoms.[9] A study done a few years earlier compared Remifemin with Premarin .625mg and Valium 2 mg in the treatment of hot flashes. Remifemin was found to be superior to both![10]

The data indicates that the most appropriate beginning dose is one tablet twice a day (20 mg per tablet). If patients have not seen significant improvement by the first month, I don't hesitate to change the dosage to two tablets twice a day. The safety of black cohosh is exceptional and has been studied and documented in over sixty years of use in Germany.[11]

Progesterone Cream

There is evidence that "natural" progesterone cream is helpful for many menopausal symptoms. I have found it most useful as an adjunct to treatment for hot flashes. Data supporting this is beginning to appear. Two papers at the recent meeting of the World Congress on Fertility and Sterility showed significant improvement in hot flashes for women using progesterone cream versus placebo. There are many anecdotal reports of its effectiveness, and I suspect that more investigations will be forthcoming. I have used it in my practice, specifically for hot flashes, and seen reasonable improvement. I use both a compounding pharmacy to make the cream (a prescription form), and several good quality over-the-counter brands, such as Angel Care, manufactured in Atlanta. The minimal concentration I use is 400 mg/oz. I then recommend a 1/4–1/2 teaspoon (~30 mg) twice a day rubbed on the abdomen, buttocks, or breast. I have also found that the progesterone cream can enhance libido . . . but only if applied by your husband!

If you use the over-the-counter progesterone cream, make sure that it actually contains progesterone. Many advertised as "wild yam cream" or "natural progesterone" actually contain the precursor of progesterone and not the actual progesterone. A woman's body cannot convert these precursor substances to progesterone, so these creams are basically worthless. If the contents label doesn't actually say progesterone, leave it alone. The dosage and frequency of use varies. It is largely a trial-and-error approach since the absorption of the cream varies in different women.

Other Approaches

Although they are not treatments in the true sense of the word, two dietary restrictions are important in reducing and eliminating hot flashes. Sometimes it is more important to eliminate aggravating factors than to treat existing symptoms. I find that women are often not aware that they may be exacerbating their problems by doing certain things. First, get rid of caffeine in your life! This powerful drug can ignite hot flashes with passion. Eliminating sodas, coffee, tea, and chocolate will help in most cases. And don't forget those caffeine-containing headache remedies.

Eliminating alcohol can also reduce hot flashes. Alcohol has been identified as a trigger for the flashes. You booze, you lose!

Stress has also been shown to be a major trigger for hot flashes. Women who are bothered by hot flashes almost universally see an exacerbation of the flashes during high-stress situations.

Several other herbs have been touted as fire extinguishers for hot flashes. These include Dong Quai, Borage seed oil, licorice root, and Motherwort Leaf. These remedies suffer the same problem as many herbal preparations—most of the information is anecdotal and word of mouth. They may work for some. However, given the high placebo response rate, it is hard to know without studies what is really doing the job. I would use proven remedies first before choosing these herbs. If the established approaches are unsuccessful, then it would be worthwhile to experiment with these second line substances.

Treatment Summary

1. Minimize stress.
2. Increase phytoestrogens in your diet or use supplments.
3. Decrease caffeine and alcohol.
4. Exercise.
5. Take vitamin E, 800 units a day minimum.
6. Try Remifemin, one to two tablets twice a day.
7. Use Progesterone cream, 1/4-1/2 teaspoon twice a day.
8. Try Tri-est tablets or cream.
9. Try estradiol (E2) tablets.

I recommend following a step-by-step approach. Start with number one and work your way down. *Everyone* can eliminate hot flashes through one or a combination of these tools.

Mood Changes, Anxiety, Depression

Moodiness, anxiety, and depression are combined (even though they are distinct clinical entities) because of the similarity of symptoms and their common response to treatments. Women have long known that there is a link between menopause and moods. Next to hot flashes, surveys show that alterations in mood are the next most common symptom of menopause. Studies report that up to 70 percent of physician office visits are anxiety-related. My experience in private practice confirms this. And I would say that was a conservative estimate. The science now exists to back up what was previously known intuitively.

There is a link between estrogen and serotonin, an important brain hormone that has a marked effect on moods. Estrogen can act as a modulator in the metabolism of this hormone, and that in turn alters emotions. The lack of estrogen also has a bearing on how serotonin is processed by the body. There is mounting evidence that the brain actually contains receptors that snatch estrogen out of the bloodstream. The research seems to be indicating that hormones influence brain chemistry much more than once thought.

Not every woman will experience behavioral changes in the menopause. Many may see subtle, temporary alterations that only they will notice. It is good to be sensitive to these changes, yet they are of such minimal consequence that they rarely warrant much intervention. The regimens discussed here are most useful to women who notice a disruption of normal functioning, a change in their ability to enjoy life, or a breakdown in interpersonal relationships. A word of caution: There are many things that can elicit such changes. Midlife is a normally stressful time. Career changes, kids leaving, kids coming back, spouses retiring—all this can impact the emotional dance through midlife.

The biggest mistake people make is attributing all the consequences to hormones. Doctors are notorious for perpetuating this myth, because it is much easier to treat someone with a pill than to listen to her talk about her broken marriage or troublesome kids. Women are perhaps worse when it comes to denial about their emotional health. "I didn't do anything about it, because I thought it was just hormones." "I'm not depressed; my hormones are just out of balance." "Yes, my husband is having an affair, but if I could just get back on track with these hormones, things would work out!" You may be giggling at these statements, but they have been sincerely spoken in my office.

So, I caution you once again: Don't wear hormone blinders. Certainly menopausal changes can elicit emotional upheavals; however, use this time to take an honest look at your stress level, your relationships, your job, other physical problems, or medications you may be taking. They can all have a marked effect on your behavior.

Melinda's Story

Melinda called me late one night. "Doc, I'm on an emotional roller coaster. One minute I am up, the next I am down. My boss says I'd better get straightened out or I may be out of a job." She is fifty-two, mother of two high school students, and a full-time secretary at a local law firm. Her story is a common one. She was concerned about the mood changes that she had begun to notice about two years ago. Her initial thoughts were: No big deal. It's just hormones. It will pass.

She began taking estrogen about a year ago and noticed the moods seemed to level out. However, over the past six months she noticed her sleep was becoming more disrupted, and her stress level was climbing. Her job was placing more demands on her; the workload had increased dramatically, while the number of people doing the work stayed the same. Her kids were, well, just teenagers. The next day in the office whe described herself as "a rubber band wound tight." She really had no other complaints other than "stuff in my head."

Melinda was experiencing many of the symptoms of overload, and the key to her feeling better was distinguishing between what was hormones and what was stress. This is often a difficult distinction. For Melinda, it turned out that it was a combination of both. So I offered her a combination of herbs and plugged into a good Christain counselor. Two months later she was actively practicing several stress management techniques and was feeling much less overburdened.

I already mentioned that ERT/HRT, because of the brain/estrogen interaction, can have a mood-elevating effect. I don't downplay the benefits that some women receive from using ERT. I vividly remember a beautiful, middle-aged woman who came into my office one month after I placed her on estradiol (E2). She gave me a gorgeous landscape painting. She said it had been years since she had felt like painting, and she didn't know why. She felt that creative spark again soon after starting on the medicine, and her low mood lifted. So, in proper context and for the right reasons, ERT can be good. My bias is to try some of the following complementary approches first.

Black Cohosh

Once again, our friend black cohosh has been shown in studies to improve mood and to treat depressive symptoms secondary to menopause. A study in 1964 had 135 patients using Remifemin, one tablet twice a day, with significant improvement in moods as measured over a two-month period. Another work published in 1987 showed a significant reduction on the Hamilton Anxiety Scale in black cohosh users as compared to placebo.[12] Remifemin, one to two tablets twice a day, over four to six weeks is a proven alternative. Just recently the company, Phytopharmica, has come out with a Remifemin Plus, which contains black cohosh and St. John's Wort. I anxiously await the research on this combined pill. Logic says it should be quite effective.

Exercise

Remember when I asked what you would do if I told you I had a pill that, taken once a day, could lift depression, reduce stress, and improve sleep? Would you take it? Well, I do, and it is called exercise! Several studies, including one in *American Psychologist* in 1981, illustrate the undeniable mental benefits of moderate exercise.[13] This should be an integral component of anyone's "feel good" prescription. Walking, swimming, aerobics—anything to get your heart rate elevated for thirty to forty minutes three times a week is good. At this ,level, more is better. I don't think most of us have to worry about overdosing on exercise.

God's creation is so miraculous that even doing something that will maximize our physical health helps us mentally. Covert Bailey, author and exercise physiologist, says, "Adaptation to exercise also produces a mental adaptation. Highly fit people usually have three personality traits: They perform well in stress/challenge tests, they exhibit emotional stability, and they are more resistant to depression and anxiety.[14]

5HTP

5-Hydroxytryptophan (5HTP) is an amino acid derivative that is important as a building block of the neurohormone serotonin. (I suspect we are going to hear a lot more in the ensuing years about serotonin and its impact on emotions.) In a study published in *Psychopathology* in 1991, 5HTP was shown to be equal to Fluvoxamine, a prescription antidepressant, in treating mild depression.[15] The patients received 100 mg of 5HTP three times a day for six weeks. The 5HTP group also reported a quicker onset of action than the Fluvoxamine patients. The side effect profile was of major importance. Patient satisfaction was higher with 5HTP, and it was better tolerated. The dosage commonly studied is 100 mg three times a day; however, the safety of much higher dosages has been assessed. 5HTP can be found in most health food stores and from reliable nutraceutical companies.

St. John's Wort

The winner of the "I am not gonna take that because of its weird name" herb award is St. John's Wort (Hypericum Perforatum). This herb has received much attention recently from the press and others. As is often the case with the media, the "facts" are often incomplete or misleading. The standardized extract of Hypericum (.3 percent Hypericin) is the most studied and scrutinized of any treatments of mood disorders in the complementary armamentarium. In a sum-mary of nine different studies compiled recently, St. John's Wort showed a decrease in depression symptoms in 59 percent of patients as compared to 20 percent in placebo use.[16] A 1994 study by Vorbach compared St. John's Wort to Imipramine, a well-known prescription antidepressant. Of 67 patients using St. John's Wort, 42 showed a positive response, whereas with the 68 patients using the Imipramine, 37 showed a positive response. St.

John's Wort was reported to have fewer side effects and better patient tolerance and acceptability.[17]

One notable side effect is increased photosensitivity (tendency to sunburn). Discontinue the herb at least two weeks before a beach vacation, or better yet, stay out of the midday rays. An excellent review article in 1996 looked at all the scientifically-sound studies done with St. John's Wort. The authors concluded from all the data that Hypericum extracts were more effective than placebo in the treat-ment of mild to moderate depression.[18]

This is not a quick fix. The average time for the onset of action for this herb is four to six weeks. However, studies confirm that persistence and consistency pay off. This is not for people who are severely depressed or suicidal. All of the studies listed here report some effectiveness for mild to moderate depression. Don't forget that the average time for improvement is four to six weeks. If you or someone you know is very down and a potential danger to themselves or others, seek immediate help. Don't experiment with herbs in this scenario.

A generally-accepted dose for effectiveness is 300 mg (.3 percent Hypericin) three times a day. Don't be misled; this is not effective as a quick fix to just "feel better." This is meant to be a long-term approach to a mild problem. Serious depression is rarely alleviated by this herb alone. Don't hesitate to consult a counselor, doctor, or pastor if you feel your depression is severe.

Ginkgo Biloba

Ginkgo is the oldest-living tree species in the world. For women over fifty, Gingko Biloba has been shown to be effective in reducing scores on the Hamilton Depression Scale, a measure of depressive feelings.[19] Interestingly these same investigators found that Ginkgo Biloba improved the effect of standard antidepressants when used together. Ginkgo has long been touted as a memory enhancer; however, most of the clinical work shows that this benefit may be limited to people over fifty. No one has been able to explain why this is specific to this age group. Animal studies suggest the mechanism of action revolves around the increase in serotonin receptors by Ginkgo.

Gingko is also known to increase blood flow in small vessels, thereby improving the symptoms of decreased blood flow to the brain, such as poor memory and confusion. A randomized, double blind, placebo-controlled study published in the *Journal of the American Medical Association* reported that Gingko Biloba extract may slow the progression of Alzheimer's disease.[20] A typical dose found to be effective is 80 mg three times a day(standardized extract). It can be combined with other herbs such as St. John's Wort. The proposed mechanism of action of Gingko would actually be synergistic and may enhance the action of both.

Stress and Anxiety

Anxiety has been called the "designer disease" of the nineties. For those in the menopause who suffer with chronic anxiety or stress related conditions, see the chapter on PMS where effective stress management techniques are discussed. I am convinced that a needed addition to any treatment for anxiety is prayer and a deep understanding that God is with you and will see you through any problem or hardship.

Often God works through others in dispelling anxiety. Of course you have to be open and accepting of that grace. God worked through Boaz in helping Ruth overcome her worry and concern about what others in the community thought about her. "Now don't worry about a thing, my daughter. I will do what is necessary, for everyone in town knows you are an honorable woman." (Ruth 3:11)

If you are stressed-out about a battle you have to fight (literally or figuratively), remember the words of puny little David going to rough up bad boy Goliath. "Don't worry about a thing," David told Saul. "I'll go fight this Philistine!" Remember that all David had on his side was God. Now He is my kind of tag team partner. And He can be yours in all your stressful battles!

Are you stressed because of the injustices in your life or in the world? Elihu thought that was job's problem, so he chastised him: "But you are too obsessed with judgment on the godless. Don't worry, justice will be upheld." (Job 36:17) It is difficult when we witness injustice. This can be a significant source of anxiety in midlife as you take stock of your life. The entire book of Job is a masterpiece on how to survive suffering and loss. Anyone who has suffered a loss or cried out "Why me?" should immerse themselves in Job and learn the peace God can give in the midst of this suffering.

The Psalmist says it best: "Don't worry about the wicked. Don't envy those who do wrong." And, "Be still in the presence of the LORD, and wait patiently for him to act. Don't worry about evil people who prosper or fret about their wicked schemes." (Psalm 37:1 and 7)

An effective tool for stress management is to stop focusing on your own problems and help someone else. This is a powerful way of shifting the emphasis from "Woe is me" to "Whoa, it's me!" The writer of Proverbs knew this as he wrote, "Worry weighs a person down; an encouraging word cheers a person up" (Proverbs 12:25). Perhaps the most illuminating advice on worry and anxiety comes from Mathew's Gospel. Jesus is talking to the people about many subjects, and he speaks directly to you and me when he says:

> So I tell you, don't worry about everyday life—whether you have enough food, drink, and clothes. Doesn't life consist of more than food and clothing? Look at the birds. They don't need to plant or harvest or put food in barns because your heavenly Father feeds them. And you are far more valuable to him than they are. Can all your worries add a single moment to your life? Of course not.
>
> And why worry about your clothes? Look at the lilies and how they grow. They don't work or make their clothing, yet Solomon in all his glory was not dressed as beautifully as they are. And if God cares so wonderfully for flowers that are here today and gone tomorrow, won't he more surely care for you? You have so little faith!
>
> So don't worry about having enough food or drink or clothing. Why be like the pagans who are so deeply concerned about these things? Your heavenly Father already knows all your needs, and he will give you all you need from day to day if you live for him and make the Kingdom of God your primary concern. So

don't worry about tomorrow, for tomorrow will bring its own worries. Today's trouble is enough for today. (Matt. 6:25–34)

Never has it been said more eloquently. This message should be shouted from the rooftops of Wall Street to the palm trees of Los Angeles. It is the ultimate hope for this anxiety-ridden world. God provides for our troubles through prayer, friends, family, fellowship, church, counseling, plants, and herbs. Don't miss the message here: These tools are acceptable to use in helping with depression or stress; they are of God. It is just as important to realize that they are only part of the picture. Being an active participant in determining your physical and emotional health is paramount. All the different tools can be utilized to achieve the balance of the healing triad: mind, body, and spirit.

Two additional herbs that have been used for anxiety are Valerian (Valeriana Officinalis) and Kava (Piper Methysticum). Valerian, a bright pink-and-white flowered rhizome native to Europe, is thought to exert its sedating effect by stimulating the release of GABA, a brain neurotransmitter.[21] It is mainly used for sleep, but I have found its calming effect helpful in chronic anxiety.

Kava is a plant indigenous to the South Sea Islands and was originally imported from there by European travelers. An interesting study in Germany in 1991 showed anxiety in menopausal women significantly improved after one week of Kava-Kava use.[22] Kava can be consumed as a beverage (as it is in the South Seas), and too much can cause over-sedation and mental impairment. This is rarely a problem with the standardized extracts in dosages of 100 mg three times a day. Kava should never be used in people with Parkinson's disease or those taking Valium or similar drugs. Don't take Kava and drive or do anything requiring quick reflexes until you determine how it will affect your system.

Treatment Summary

1. Pray, immerse yourself in the Word, and call on God for help.
2. Exercise, three times a week for thirty to forty minutes (ideally every day).

3. Try St. John's Wort, 300 mg three times a day (don't take if you are already on an antidepressant).
4. Take 5HTP, 100 mg three times a day.
5. If over fifty, take Gingko Biloba, 80 mg three times a day.
6. Talk to a Christian counselor.
7. Some may benefit from traditional antidepressant treatment; don't rule it out!

Insomnia and Fatigue

One of the most common complaints of the menopause is a lack of restful sleep. Like many other problems insomnia can have a multitude of causes. It is important, as with treating any of these problems, to work in concert with a trusted, competent medical professional to make sure that there are no other underlying problems. Again, don't fall into the trap of wearing blinders when it comes to menopausal symptoms.

I have included fatigue in this category because one of the leading causes of energy drain in this population is poor sleep. They go hand in hand and seem to set up a repetitive cycle. Lack of sleep leads to tiredness the next day. This in turn leads to disrupted sleep the next night and the cycle repeats. Eventually the sleeplessness is manifested as overall fatigue and moodiness. As an obstetrician, I have firsthand experience with the effects of sleep deprivation. Babies just don't understand office hours.

There is ample evidence that many of the sleep problems of the menopause arise from the disruptive nature of hot flashes. Many women experience an increase in hot flashes at night. We are not sure why this happens, but some feel it is a response of the hypothalamus to the decreased activity of the body during the night hours. It's as if the brain gets bored and says, "Hey, let's make this gal miserable and keep her up at night."

The obvious first approach to aiding sleep is to get rid of the hot flashes. This really isn't rocket science! See the section on hot flashes for a guaranteed successful approach.

What if you have eliminated the night sweats (or never had them) and still have problems sleeping? What options are available other than potentially addictive sleeping pills? Again I must say emphatically that you have to be sure that no other problems exist that may be influencing your sleep. Many maladies, ranging from thyroid disorders to psychiatric conditions, can alter normal sleep. You must address those problems. Be sure you are not just treating symptoms and not causes. A stress-filled day does not make for a relaxing night. Psalm 77:4 says, "You don't let me sleep. I am too distressed even to pray!"

Identify any predisposing factors such as anxiety, medications you may be taking, or physical symptoms such as pain. Eliminate those before assuming your problem with sleep is strictly menopause-related.

God has provided many "natural" sleep aids that have proven effectiveness. God told the Israelites, "I will give you peace in the land, and you will be able to sleep without fear" (Leviticus 26:6). A peaceful heart and mind allow for a fearless sleep. "People who work hard sleep well, whether they eat little or much. But the rich are always worrying and seldom get a good night's sleep." (Prov. 20:13) The writer of Proverbs makes two important points about sleep in this verse. First, we know anecdotally and scientifically that exercise improves sleep. The Israelites knew it a long time ago. (For them it was not called exercise; it was called work.) If you are having a problem sleeping, get off your rear end and get active! It can't hurt, and it will help! That doesn't mean running a mile before bed. That would have just the opposite effect. But a healthy amount of activity during the day definitely promotes sleep. The second point made in the above verse is not that poor people sleep better than rich people, but that anxiety and worry are a leading cause of sleeplessness.

Sleepy-Time Herbs

What are some natural approaches to sleep? 5-Hydroxytryptophan, or 5HTP, has been seen in several double-blind studies to decrease the number of nighttime awakenings. A work published in 1988 reports that 5HTP not only aids in quantity of sleep but also in quality. The amount of REM, or rapid eye movement sleep, which is the most restful, increased.[23]

Valerian Root (Valeriana Officinalis) has been used for many years as a sedative and sleep aid. In 1982, a study was published that showed that Valerian was able to improve the perceived quality of sleep in self-reported poor sleepers.[24] This was confirmed in 1989 in a study where 89 percent reported improved sleep with the use of Valerian.[25] A major plus for the use of Valerian is the apparent lack of daytime drowsiness that can be associated with a traditional sleeping pill. The standard dose used in these studies is 1 to 3 grams about thirty minutes before bed. Be careful with Valerian. If used properly and in appropriate doses it can be effective; however, it should not be used with any other prescription sleeping aids or benzodiazapines.

The best-known alternative sleep aid is melatonin. Melatonin is a hormone secreted by the pineal gland, a small gland in the base of the brain. Unfortunately this hormone has been tainted by misinformation and media hype. There are a lot of shady operators and con men and women in the "natural" medicine field, and none more so than in the promotion of melatonin. There is no question that melatonin has been shown to be a wonderful sleep aid, but only in people who have a low melatonin level.[26] Melatonin taken by people with normal levels (and that is the vast majority of us) will do little if anything for sleep, and may even backfire and disrupt sleep patterns. Women over the age of sixty have a higher likelihood of low melatonin, so they may experience some benefit from the substance. Before using this, see your doctor and be evaluated for its potential for effectiveness.

Some women suffer from leg cramping that keeps them awake at night. One suggestion that has worked in my practice is bedtime magnesium tablets in a dose of 250-500 mg.

Treatment Summary

1. Reduce stress.
2. Eliminate hot flashes.
3. Exercise.

4. Take 5HTP, 100 mg three times a day.
5. Use Valerian Root extract, 1–3 grams one-half hour before bed.
6. Try melatonin, if a deficiency exists.
7. Try estradiol (E2) or Tri-est.

Libido

Sex drive, or libido, is one of the most complex of human behaviors. Some studies estimate that only a fraction of women actually suffer from hormone-induced decreased libido. By that I mean that there are few instances where a decreased sex drive is due solely to menopause. This may not be a popular stance, yet science supports the idea that hormones play a relatively small role in sex drive. Energy level, stress, mental discord, and past history all play a significant role in determining libido. Since these are all individual experiences, it follows that sex drive is rarely the same for two people.

In a recent survey, 35 percent of menopausal women said their sex life was actually better than before, whereas 25 percent said it was about the same. What may constitute normality for one may be viewed as decreased by another. However, there is no denying that there is a distinct role, albeit minimal, that hormones play in influencing sex drive. This role can be primary or secondary, particularly with menopausal women.

It is primary in that there is a connection between decreasing estrogen and progesterone, and possibly testosterone, and decreased libido; and secondary in that declining estrogen may lead to thinning of the vaginal and vulvar skin, which in turn leads to pain or discomfort with intercourse. It is a simple deduction that if it hurts, you avoid it!

Estradiol Cream

An obvious solution to the dyspareunia (painful intercourse) is to replenish those tissues and stop the pain. Once this is accomplished, libido commonly improves. The most effective way of improving vaginal dryness and increasing lubrication is with the use of estradiol preparations. The scientific studies confirm this as the unquestionable leader in vaginal lining stimulation. The radical "naturalists" will just have to grin and bear this one because the research shows that there are some complementary approaches to vaginal dryness, but they are not as effective as estrogen cream.

I feel confident about this recommendation because, except for the occasional breast tenderness, the side effects are minimal. There is very little absorption into the bloodstream, so the systemic risks are minimized. I prefer estradiol cream to the conjugated estrogens simply because of its single estrogen content. The creams have an advantage for the vagina because they deliver the active ingredient directly to the tissues in need. An interesting product recently made available is a small flexible ring embedded with estradiol that fits in the vagina and gives a slow release of the hormone over several months. Some women like this because it eliminates the mess of the creams. Others object to the idea of any thing foreign staying in the vaginal canal for that length of time. It is a personal preference. I have found that many women on oral hormone preparations often experience vaginal dryness and painful intercourse in spite of adequate doses.

All is not lost for the purists who are die-hard estrogen haters; there are other options for improving vaginal lubrication and libido. Vitamin E gel or liquid has been shown to improve vaginal skin thickness and lubrication. I tell patients to take the 1,000 mg capsules and poke a hole in them and then rub the oil in the vaginal canal and on the labia twice a day. Remifemin, the standardized dose of black cohosh, has been effective in promoting normal lubrication.[27] Dr. John Lee, in his book *What Your Doctor May Not Tell You about Menopause*, claims that "natural progesterone" cream can relieve vaginal atrophy.

There are several over-the-counter lubricant products that have been helpful in treating this bothersome condition. Lubrin and Replens are two that are commonly available. They are nonhormonal and work with your body's own moisture to promote lubrication.

Here is something you may or may not want to hear. Increasing the frequency of intercourse can actually improve vaginal dryness! Is God great or what? He has designed the body to work better if it is used more often. Now that is a nice piece of engineering! This knowledge is for women only. I'll never forget the lady who, with all seriousness, asked me for a note that said she didn't have to have sex for three months. Not a common or healthy request! You don't have to share this news with your husband if you don't want to. Your secret is safe with me!

Don't forget to check the medicines that you take. Antihistamines and diuretics can dry the mucus membranes (and the vaginal lining) and should be avoided if possible. Also remember to increase your dietary intake of phytoestrogens.

Other Options

Now that we have conquered the vaginal problem (that sounds ominous doesn't it?), let's look at some other ways to enhance libido. Testosterone has long been identified as the hormone that seems to exert a stimulating effect on sexual desire. This is especially apparent in women who have had their ovaries removed at the time of hysterectomy. Because the ovaries are the primary source of testosterone in the female and because they continue to produce testosterone into the menopause, the use of testosterone is becoming more popular as a component of HRT. Studies are conclusive that testosterone supplementation can enhance libido to a degree, and they have also been credited with producing a general sense of well-being. Recent work also points out that the use of androgens (testosterone) in the menopause may have a positive effect on lessening bone loss.[28]

However, as with all medicines, there are side effects and risks. One of the most common and most disturbing side effects is increased hair growth, and I am not talking about on the head. Actually some women have reported hair loss from their heads! In various cases some have had deepening of the voice, weight gain, enlargement of the clitoris, oily skin, and acne.

Probably the biggest potential concern with testosterone use is the effect on the blood lipids. Some studies suggest that testosterone increases the triglyceride levels and has a minimal effect on the total cholesterol (may be a slight decrease in HDL values).

Recent work states that the addition of low-dose androgens to a standard HRT regimen will not significantly decrease its otherwise beneficial effect on heart disease.[29] Studies are continuing, and the definitive word will be forthcoming. Compounding pharmacies can make a testosterone cream that produces lower blood levels than the oral testosterone and avoids some of the bothersome side effects. I have read a few studies that report libido enhancement with the cream. Patients in my practice have had success with a 2–5 percent cream rubbed on the abdomen twice a day. Once again, with the use of testosterone, either solely or in conjunction with other substances, you must look at the benefit/risk ratio or, in partnership with a knowledgeable health care person, make a decision based solely on your needs. In addition, testosterone may be administered in shots or pellets, yet the side effects are usually more pronounced because of the increased blood levels.

Many herbal products have been touted through the years as aphrodisiacs. Most of these are just fantasy and rely on the placebo effect for any benefit. Siberian ginseng, for example, has been long touted for its sexual enhancement ability. A search of the literature revealed only three studies that attempted to speak to this scientifically, and two of those were done on bulls! I can't recommend the use of ginseng in this capacity unless you own impotent bulls!

Communication

Finally, one of the most important things to focus on in enhancing libido is good communication with your husband. Talking about each other's sexuality, needs, wants, and problems can eliminate many misunderstandings. I have seen couples who realize separately there is a problem, yet they never discuss it. This in turn develops into many false assumptions that can be quite damaging. These misperceptions easily lead to festering sores that can eat away at a relationship. You must bring up the issue, if for no other reason than to acknowledge it exists. Many women relate that they didn't think they had a problem until their husband said they did! Rarely is it the other way around.

This leads to the point that many struggle with. What is normal? Sexologists have debated this for years, and I suspect will continue to, for this question is unanswerable.

Essentially, normal is what is normal for you. What is your baseline? What feels right to you? Often I tell women that a change in libido is much more significant than someone who has "always" had a low sexual appetite. And remember that, because God has made you different from your spouse, your individual sexual desires may vary tremendously. If that is the case, then your idea of "normal" is really based on your own experience and not the feelings of your partner. Determining what is normal for you as a couple takes some discussion and honest evaluation of your differences. Then the task is to take these differences and blend them into the relationship in healthy ways that nourish both partners. Don't get caught in the trap of feeling you "need" some libido help without first going through this process.

Treatment Summary

1. Reduce stress and fatigue (two leading causes of decreased sex drive).
2. Explore relationship issues and discuss them with your husband. Sex is often a mirror of the health of the relationship.
3. Eliminate vaginal dryness with vitamin E, Remifemin, HRT, vaginal inserts, and estrogen creams.
4. Use testosterone cream 2–5 percent, 1/2 tsp. once or twice a day.
5. If you are on HRT, consider adding testosterone to the regimen (after evaluation).

Urinary Complaints

"Every time I cough I wet my pants."

"I can't sing in the choir anymore because hitting the high notes means changing underwear."

"If I don't go right when I feel the urge, watch out. It's trouble."

"Even after I go I feel like I haven't fully emptied my bladder."

These statements are all too common in the postmenopausal woman. Estimates say that over 13 million women in the United States are incontinent. That translates into 33 percent of the population! What is staggering is that 50–70 percent of those affected don't tell their doctor about their problem and don't seek help. It is estimated that the health costs because of incontinence amount to 20 billion dollars a year.

The message is twofold. One, you are not alone. Most people don't go to cocktail parties and sit around and say, "So, Marge, how is the dribbling?" It is a subject that is not talked about, but chances are someone close to you has a problem with urinary incontinence. Many women don't discuss it with their doctor because they are embarrassed, or they think nothing can be done, or they don't want any surgery, or they feel it is a normal sign of aging. Poppycock to all those excuses!

Two, there is a lot that can be done for urinary incontinence both surgically and nonsurgically. Understanding the physiology helps to understand the options. Urinary incontinence consists of four basic types: (1) anatomical droppage of the bladder—stress incontinence, (2) bladder spasms—detrusor instability, (3) a mixture of the two-the most common, and (4) overflow incontinence. Overflow incontinence is mainly limited to women with diabetes or selective neurological problems, and since it is relatively rare I won't spend much time discussing this type.

Stress incontinence is due to an anatomical drop in the bladder and is secondary to childbirth, aging, and loss of hormonal stimulation of the bladder and urethra, or a prior hysterectomy. It is treated in a variety of ways, but the majority involves a surgical correction of the bladder position (bladder tack). Contrast this with a bladder spasm, which is treated mainly with behavioral modification and medication. Thus you can see identifying the type of incontinence is vital to be able to choose the most effective treatment. Doing a bladder tack for bladder spasms will still leave you wet, and treating stress incontinence with medications will not solve that problem. The third category mentioned is a combination of both, and some estimates state that 60–75 percent of incontinent women have this mixture.

You must distinguish which type of incontinence is the predominant one. This will guide your therapy options. If you have a problem that is predominately bladder spasms, you should achieve adequate control from some medications and bladder retraining and never entertain the thought of surgery.

Why is this important? Because a substantial number of women in the menopause suffer with incontinence. One of the first things women can do for this problem is assess their hormonal status. The bladder and urethra are hormone-sensitive tissues, and urgency and incontinence may arise simply from a lack of estrogen stimulation. Many women use some form of estrogen (creams, pills, etc.) and a few months later their bladder troubles markedly improve. It certainly is worth discussing with your doctor as part of your evaluation.

There are other methods to thwart stress urinary incontinence. One of the most useful is an exercise for the bladder. (I know you think I'm obsessed with exercise.) Many of you may already be familiar with Kegel exercises. When used consistently and persistently, they work! I have seen women avoid surgery and maintain continence from doing these simple exercises. The two biggest mistakes women make are doing the exercises wrong or not being persistent enough.

Next time you are sitting on the commode, consciously stop your stream. The muscles that you tighten are the muscles that you want to exercise. The idea is to contract these muscles and hold them for five seconds and then relax, and then repeat. Do this for five minutes three times a day, and I guarantee you will see the benefits after a month. Have fun with it. The wonderful thing about this exercise is no one knows you are doing anything. There are no special clothes to buy, no special machines needed, and you will never be annoyed by 30-minute infomercials about them! Associate with something to help you remember to do the Kegels. For example, every time the phone rings, do your Kegels! (Use something different if you are a secretary or receptionist, or you may end up with a muscle-bound bladder!) It is not quick, but it will work. The other alternatives are (1) to live with it, and (2) to pay for a surgeon's new car.

A related, yet separate topic is cystitis, or bladder infection. This common female problem seems to be accentuated during the menopause. This is largely due to the change in the normally acidic vaginal contents to a more basic environment. This in turn leads to alteration in the type and amount of bacteria in the vaginal canal. Because of the close anatomical relationship between the urethra and the vagina, it is easy for bacteria to migrate into the bladder where they are not welcome. This is the reason why intercourse is a predisposing cause of frequent bladder infections for some women. In the menopause, because of decreasing lubrication, some women experience a rise in the frequency of cystitis. There are some effective ways of not only treating these infections but also of preventing infections from ever bothering you.

First and foremost, you must drink adequate amounts of fluid. Drink a minimum of six to eight glasses a day. This is but a baseline; active people require much more. Water is the best, but cranberry juice is helpful, especially for the bladder. Initially scientists speculated that it was the acid nature of the cranberry juice that exerted its protective effect; however, studies have shown that it is actually a substance in the juice that has antiseptic properties. This again is one of those old wives tales that has been proven true by legitimate scientific studies. A work done in 1991 published in the prestigious *New England Journal of Medicine* examined the beneficial effect of unsweetened cranberry juice and concluded it was effective at decreasing the frequency of urinary tract infections.[30]

Two other complementary approaches to preventing bladder infections involve the herb Uva-Ursi (sounds like a constellation) and Goldenseal. In 1993, Larsson and colleagues used 250 mg of Uva-Ursi in 57 women with documented frequent urinary tract infections. The amazing results were that no women in the treatment group suffered a bout of cystitis for an entire year ![31]

Goldenseal has long been known for its antibiotic-like effects. A study published in 1969 documented that the berberine in Goldenseal was effective in treating uncomplicated urinary tract infections.[32] A word of caution, bladder infections by themselves are usually pretty harmless except for the discomfort they cause. However, if they go untreated or improperly treated they could progress to a more serious infection. If you are using complementary methods of treating your cystitis, don't hesitate to contact your health care provider if you are not seeing improvement in your symptoms within 48 hours. Complementary approaches are much more effective in preventing cystitis than treating it.

Treatment Summary

1. Discuss it with your doctor, as it can't be helped if it is ignored.
2. Identify the type of incontinence (hard to do by yourself, see above).
3. Consider estradiol or estriol cream.
4. Eliminate caffeine.
5. Do Kegel exercises.
6. Use surgical correction as last resort for anatomical incontinence.

Headaches, Joint Aches, Body Aches

Laura was a bright, athletic woman in her late forties. She was menopausal, having stopped her periods one year prior. I remembered her especially because she, like me, was an avid distance runner. It would not be unusual for her to run thirty to forty miles a week. She had just finished her fourth marathon when she came for a routine checkup. Menopause had been little more than a blip on her screen, as she had experienced an occasional hot flash and that was it.

On this visit she said she was doing great except she was noticing some achiness in her wrists and shoulders. It wasn't severe, and she described it as a deep type of discomfort that didn't keep her from doing things (obviously), but was nagging. I initially wrote it off as being a residual effect from her recent marathon. I told her to get plenty of rest and decrease her mileage over the next month. If i didn't get better, come and see me then. A month passed, and I had forgotten our discussion when I saw her running on the riverbank one Saturday morning. We ran together for a while, and she said she had fully recovered from the race and was only doing two to three mile runs, but the discomfort she had described earlier was still there. From her description I suspected an orthopedic problem so I set up a referral with a colleague the next week.

I spoke to her a few weeks later and found out that he had put her through a whole battery of tests and could find nothing to explain her pain. She was taking Motrin and it helped, but she was concerned that she was treating a symptom and not a cause.

It just so happened that I had spent the previous weekend in Atlanta at a conference on complementary approaches to common health problems, and one of the presenters had talked about "body ache, bone pain" syndrome of menopause. He stated that many women will experience this nonspecific ache in any bone or joint in the body, and this was thought to be secondary to the decreased lubrication and secretions of the joint space. This sounded amazingly like Laura's situation, so when I got back I called her and discussed what I had learned. The first thing we did was to increase her dietary phytoestrogens. Then we added some Tri-est cream. Within two weeks she was noticing some improvement, but she didn't feel we were there yet.

I then suggested glucosamine sulfate. Glucosamine is a naturally occurring substance that plays an important role in the biochemistry of cartilage; in particular it serves as the basic building block of glycosaminoglycans that are essential components of cartilage. Glucosamine sulfate has been studied extensively in treating osteoarthritis, and has been shown to have an anti-inflammatory effect. A large multicentered trial in France compared the efficacy of glucosamine with that of a prescription nonsteroidal anti-inflammatory medicine, Piroxicam. They found that glucosamine was significantly more effective than the Piroxicam and placebo in relief of joint pain.[33] The presenter at this conference had taken this data and used the glucosamine in his menopausal women with these diffuse, nebulous joint discomforts. His results were impressive, so I felt it was worth a try with Laura.

Within a month she was pain free, and running better than ever! Since then, I have used this regimen and found it to be very helpful in almost everyone with these particular "achy" complaints. The most tested dose is 500 mg three times a day. Studies have also documented the safety and lack of significant side effects. The literature is full of reports of glucosamine sulfate and its potent analgesic effects, especially on bone and joint pain. Get a proper physical, and if all else appears normal, consider this wonderful solution.

Treatment Summary

1. Rule out other medical conditions.
2. Take glucosamine sulfate for joint and bone pain (500 mg three times a day).
3. Exercise.
4. Increase dietary phytoestrogens.
5. Try therapeutic massage.

SECTION FOUR

Bouncing, Binging, Bones, and Believing

CHAPTER TEN

Exercise: Sweating with the Oldies

Exercise is not an option! Immutable Rule 3: If you don't use it, you're going to lose it!

The third A in the prescription for success in menopause is action. If your goal is to live a healthy, long, happy life, exercise is not a maybe! It must be a part of your daily routine. There are multitudes of benefits, and the intensity and duration to achieve these benefits can be adapted to almost any situation.

What else can help you feel better, look better, act better, lower cholesterol, reduce fat, strengthen your heart, decrease osteoporosis, improve PMS, treat depression, boost the immune system, increase libido, improve sleep, build self-esteem—and is cheap? There is nothing else on the planet that can accomplish all this with no side effects. God has designed the perfect fountain of youth, and it is available to all regardless of age or current health. But you have to drink from it for thirty to forty-five minutes daily for it to work.

God designed us to move. Every muscle, bone, and tendon, is geared for motion. The rewards of inactivity include obesity, breathlessness, multiple medications, and depression. Proverbs 19:24 says.

"Some people are so lazy that they won't even lift a finger to feed themselves." Not a good exercise plan or weight loss diet.

The choice is yours!

Exercise Is Biblical

The Bible, especially the New Testament, is filled with analogies to athletics and physical activities. Paul's letters in particular employ physical activity imagery to drive home important spiritual points. I think it is intentional that these references appear frequently, and they underscore the importance of exercise in a balanced lifestyle. Paul writes in Corinthians,

> Remember that in a race everyone runs, but only one person gets the prize. You also must run in such a way that you will win. All athletes practice strict self-control. They do it to win a prize that will fade away, but we do it for an eternal prize. So I run straight to the goal with purpose in every step. I am not like a boxer who misses his punches. I discipline my body like an athlete, training it to do what it should. Otherwise, I fear that after preaching to others I myself might be disqualified. (Cor. 9:24–27)

Philippians 3:14 says, "I strain to reach the end of the race and receive the prize for which God, through Christ Jesus, is calling us up to heaven." In 2 Timothy 4:7, Paul writes, "I have fought a good fight, I have finished the race, and I have remained faithful. And now the prize awaits me-the crown of righteousness that the Lord, the righteous judge, will give me on that great day of His return. And the prize is not just for me but for all who eagerly look forward to His glorious return." And Hebrews 12:1 says, "Therefore, since we are surrounded by such a huge crowd of witnesses to the life of faith, let us strip off every weight that slows us down, especially the sin that so easily hinders our progress. And let us run with endurance the race that God has set before us."

I have no doubt that Paul had spent time walking and running on the fields and hills of the Holy Land on many a bright morning!

MARATHON

A verse that inspired me and helped me survive my first marathon was Isaiah 40:28–31:

> Have you never heard or understood? Don't you know that the LORD is the everlasting God, the Creator of all the earth? He never grows faint or weary. No one can measure the depths of His understanding. He gives power to those who are tired and worn out; He offers strength to the weak. Even youths will become exhausted, and young men will give up. But those who wait on the LORD will find new strength. They will fly high on wings like eagles. They will run and not grow weary. They will walk and not faint.

This was my prayer as I rounded the turn and entered the final six miles of the twenty-six-mile race on the hills of San Francisco. I am convinced that without this verse to motivate me, I may not have completed that run. So it is in any endeavor. Whether it is a running race, a decision, an emotional heartbreak, or a mental challenge, God is there to provide motivation and guidance. I repeated this verse hundreds of times in my training runs and in the actual race.

Paul puts exercise in perspective in his letter to Timothy: "Physical exercise has some value, but spiritual exercise is much more important, for it promises a reward in both this life and the next" (1 Timothy 4:8). There is no question that physical exercise is beneficial, yet the focus is balance. You can let exercise (or any obsession) be an idol. Balance mind, body, and spirit.

Daily, I hear, "But, Doc, I don't have time to exercise!" Translated this really means, "I don't want to make time to exercise." Every time a patient uses, that excuse, I make a bet with her. Her visit will be free if I can't find thirty minutes in her daily schedule in which she can undertake some form of useful exercise. And I tell women I will not ask them to do anything that I won't or haven't done myself. I haven't given away a single office visit yet. (My office manager cringes every time I do this.)

I also frequently hear, "But, Doc, I'm seventy and have never exercised, what good will it do me now?"

The answer is simple—a great deal. If your doctor says you can, (and I would question him/her if they said otherwise) there is much to be gained from an exercise regimen tailored to your needs and abilities. If you are a charter member of the couch potato club, don't walk out the door tomorrow and run two miles. There is a fine line between enthusiasm and stupidity. Get proper advice from your doctor about what you can do (focus on that instead of what you can't do) and start slow. In this instance being a turtle is much more advantageous than being a rabbit. But the message is, "Just do it." Do something. Start today!

Maya Angelou said, "Lift up your hearts. Each new hour holds new chances for new beginnings." If it is no more than chair aerobics, do something. The shelves are full of good manuals on everything from Tai Chi to power walking. Get a good check up, pick something you like doing, and for your sake, do it!

An exercise regimen must be individualized. Just because Uncle Harry ran his first marathon at sixty-five doesn't mean you have to match him step for step. It also doesn't mean you can't! Again, focus on what you can do, not what restrictions you have. Too many times people begin by asking, "What are the things I shouldn't be doing." The real question is, what *can* I do?

Age Is No Barrier

You are never too old to exercise. I kid my wife when I tell her my last exercise will be pushing up daisies. Marjorie Newlin began weight lifting at age seventy-two. Her story was told in a recent *Parade* magazine article. By age seventy-eight she had accumulated twenty-five bodybuilding trophies! Not bad for a grandmother of four who began lifting weights to be able to handle everyday tasks. She started slowly, and steadily built to a level that not only wins her contests but also keeps her healthy in mind and body. Marjorie is but one of many examples of older individuals who have dramatically affected their quality of life through exercise.

A study published a few years back looked at ninety-year-old men and their ability to benefit from weight-bearing exercise. These were folks in various levels of health, and they were guided through individualized routines for six weeks. Universally the men showed improvement in strength and muscle mass. They all said they felt and slept better. One fellow said it had revived his sex life! The message is, excuses don't work, and age is not a limiting factor. The only limiting factor is the muscle between your ears!

Bob Hope once said that middle age is when your age starts to show around your middle! If that is the case, then exercise is your best middle age makeover.

If you haven't noticed by now, I believe very strongly in educating yourself about your body. The more you know, the better you take care of it. Learning basic facts of exercise and metabolism is important because it is critical to your understanding of the benefits that will be realized.

What happens when you exercise? Why is all this stuff helpful? How can I amaze and bedazzle my friends at parties with my knowledge of physiology? The answers are simple.

Fat

Fat, blubber, jelly belly, love handles, spare tire, thunder thighs—all identify the same condition, obesity. We can all agree that fat is a problem for most of us. Well, fat is actually your friend! The only problem is that most of us get too much of a good thing. You have heard of overstaying your welcome. When it comes to fat, many of us have allowed the guests to move in permanently!

Fat was deliberately put in our bodies by the good Lord not as punishment, but as a phenomenal energy source. When we spend time exercising we begin to tell the fat cells to give up some of that important fuel. After about twenty or thirty minutes of exercise the muscles scream for more energy, and the wise body responds by dipping into the fat reserves for its highly concentrated and efficient source of fuel. We "release the grease" as Covert Bailey says in his book *Smart Exercise*.

To put it simply, if we act in short bursts (like chasing the two-year-old around the house, or doing the laundry), we tend to selectively burn sugar (glucose). This sugar is readily available and easily metabolized, so it is the first choice when the activity is relatively short lived. However, if the energy expenditure extends over a longer period of time, the body calls on its reserves, fat, and begins to burn this for fuel. When fat is metabolized, miracle upon miracles, your thighs get smaller and your belly becomes flatter!

The secret to efficient fat burning is making the exercise *aerobic* and *sustained*. Aerobic means with oxygen, and this element is absolutely essential in the metabolism of fat. Your level of fitness is literally how well your muscles burn oxygen. A simple way of determining whether your exercise is aerobic is to measure your pulse while exercising, and if it is elevated above 110, you are doing something right. However, and this is just as important, you should always be able to carry on a conversation while exercising. If you are too out of breath to do this, you have to slow down and build up to that level more slowly. I run alone most times, and every now and then I will carry on a mock conversation to test whether I am going too fast. This easy to do, and it provides entertainment for those around me! Many people avoid me on purpose, and I hear them whisper, "There is the wacko who always talks to himself!"

The second component to fat-burning aerobic exercise is sustained activity. Studies show that to attain maximal fat burning you must exercise aerobically for a minimum of twenty minutes. Notice I said fat burning. There are many things that you can do that will build strength, protect bones, and contribute to overall health other than aerobic exercise. Weight lifting is rarely an aerobic exercise, but it can be very beneficial to women in the menopause, especially when dealing with osteoporosis prevention. Yoga, stretching, and Tai Chi are great exercises, yet they are rarely aerobic.

To achieve overall health for your body, consider alternating activities. This common practice, called cross training, is the quickest, most enjoyable way of achieving fitness and staying that way. For example, on Monday go for a brisk forty-five-minute walk. Tuesday spend a half-hour lifting weights. Wednesday play golf (no carts and walk fast). Thursday do yoga or stretching. Friday take another good walk. Saturday can be a second weight session, and Sunday you rest and thank God for letting you do all that stuff during the week!

The Secret to Weight Loss

Some eternal truths are painful to acknowledge. One of those is that when you take in more calories than you burn up, you gain weight. When you burn up more than you take in, you lose weight. This is a basic rule of nature, like "What goes up must come down." This is a reality of the physical world. It is unalterable regardless of the imagery or positive thinking employed. Positive thinking may help your attitude, but it won't change your fitness level.

Billions of dollars are spent each year instructing people on the best ways of losing weight. When you break down every single method to its core, it is either a way of decreasing intake (diet) or increasing output (exercise). Even all the medications available are geared to either help you eat less or attempt to fool your body into burning up more. No matter how fancy the name or how sophisticated the machine, all weight control plans fall into one of these two categories.

Let me make an important distinction. There is a common misperception that there is a relationship between being thin and being healthy. That is not the case. I know many sick skinny people and several chubby healthy folks. Granted there is more of a likelihood of medical problems in an obese woman; however, the gauge of her health does not solely depend on her bathroom scales. Health is much more than simply the absence of disease. Remember, it is a joyful balance. So a person's body contour doesn't necessarily make an accurate statement about their state of health. For example, I would much rather be twenty pounds overweight and leading an active lifestyle than at ideal body weight and smoke a pack of cigarettes a day. It is easy to equate weight with health; it's so visual! Dress size is only part of the equation. Exercise is a vital component in weight loss, and its overall benefits are much broader and far reaching.

Overweight Versus Overfat

To tie the idea of weight, health, and fat together, consider the difference between being overweight and overfat. "What is the difference?" you say. "They seem like the same thing to me."

The difference is that you can be overfat and be normal weight! For you nonexercisers this is a scary concept. Take Eloise, a forty-two-year-old woman who is 5'8" and weighs 128 lbs. She has worn the same size dress since college. She is proud that she can still wear her cheerleading outfit from high school (although I don't know why she'd want to). The problem with Eloise is not her weight but her body fat. When she was eighteen she was extremely active and exercised excessively. She weighed about 128 then, but if you compared the amount of muscle that made up her weight, you would have found that about 78 percent of her weight was lean body mass (muscle). This gave her about 22 percent body fat. This is considered very healthy for women. As she aged, Eloise became less active and her muscle mass declined. If you look at unused muscles under the microscope, you can actually see little fat cells that become deposited in the muscle. So after several years of decreased activity, Eloise now is still at 128 lbs., but her body fat has climbed to 42 percent. This leads to a corresponding drop in her lean body mass (muscle).

Stealth Obesity

Why is this important? Many people will become overfat and not realize the risk to their health. It is stealth obesity. It is there, but it is not detected before the damage is done. Many will become overfat before they become overweight.

Being overfat is responsible for increasing risk factors for heart disease, stroke, diabetes, and obesity. If you can avoid being overfat then you can avoid many of the health problems that are associated with external obesity. If you are overweight, it is something you can see, (all too well) and something you can feel and touch. It is only natural to identify visible obesity as the bad guy. Well, it is, but it is down the line from the source. If you really want to make a difference, you need to focus on how to become unfat! That is going to the source, the origin of the problem. That is solving the problem at its beginning. The goal is to be healthy, not just thin.

How do you get unfat, or ideally, prevent yourself from ever getting fat in the first place? You guessed it! Exercise. (See how all this ties together?) Exercise is not only for losing weight. My hope is that you eliminate the fixation most Americans have with weight. The goal of exercise is to get your body moving as God meant you to, and to provide an internal environment that is optimal.

The external appearance is a nice by-product, but your focus should be on the inside. When Paul said in his letter to Timothy, "Physical exercise has some value, but spiritual exercise is much more important, for it promises a reward in both this life and the next," he was making the point that what is in your heart and soul is more important than your outward appearance. This specifically applies to exercise also, in that it is not necessarily the outward appearance that is the trophy; it is the internal change that holds the promise for health and longevity. At the most basic level, exercise improves both physical and mental health. All can benefit from exercise. Thin, thick, young, old, male, female-all have a need to "Just do it."

Percent Body Fat

No doubt you all have seen the charts explaining ideal body weight. These charts have done about as much disservice to the population as the media's glamorization of the "ideal woman." The charts are inaccurate reminders of an inappropriate measurement of health. Body weight is not the best parameter to follow if you are truly interested in health. Weight is easy to measure, and there is a correlation between risk factors and weight. So in that respect the charts are peripherally useful. But given a choice, knowing your percent body fat is a much more valuable tool in assessing your health. Unfortunately it is much more difficult to get accurate measurements of body fat percentage than weight.

The best way to check your body fat is to be weighed in a water tank while submerged. The underwater immersion test is the most accurate measure, and it is the method used most often by universities and physiology labs when doing research. Not many of us can drive down the street to our friendly immersion tank and get our body fat calculated once a month, so several other methods of estimating body fat percentage have been developed.

Covert Bailey, in *Smart Exercise*, talks about a simple method you can use at your next swimming party. It's based on the fact that fat floats and muscle sinks. Have all your guests float on their backs in the pool. Have them take a deep breath and when prompted blow it all out. His informal research has shown that above 25 percent body fat, people float easily. At 22–23 percent fat, one can float while breathing shallowly. At 15 percent body fat, one will usually sink slowly even with the lungs full of air. At 13 percent body fat, one will sink readily with a chest full of air, even in salt water![1] This is a fun way to get a basic idea of body fat.

A more accurate determination is using skin calipers. It is a small, simple device that a trained person can use to grasp a skin fold, say in your upper arm, and measure the thickness. A formula can then be used to calculate the correct percent. If done properly, this can be an amazingly accurate measure of your body fat percentage. Many doctors offer these measurements in their offices, and most health clubs and gyms have someone on staff who can perform this quick and easy test. Several machines that check bone density can also assess total body fat. Next time you go in for a bone densiometry ask about getting your body fat assessed. It is not your weight, but your body fat that is important to know and follow.

Here are the important points about exercise. First, it is a must. Second, all ages and experience levels can participate. Third, when coupled with the right foods, exercise is the best way to internal health. Fourth, it can actually be fun!

Where Do I Start?

OK, so you are convinced that exercise is a good thing. "Well, Exercise Boy," you ask, "Where do I start?" For those whose idea of exercise is using the TV remote control, the place to start is with your doctor. Before you begin any new activity it is a grand idea to get a good checkup to know your starting point. Ask your doctor for guidelines. Ask how to start and what exercises would be good for you. If your doctor says you can't do at least some form of exercise, I would get a second opinion.

Almost everyone can begin a walking program. There are some obvious exceptions, but there are even options for those who can't walk. I have found through experience and the research of others that walking is one of the best forms of exercise. Start slowly, and gradually build up both miles and speed. Remember the importance of aerobic exercise to help eliminate fat. To be aerobic, exercise must be swift enough to elevate your heart rate, but not so fast that you can't continue to have a conversation while walking. This level of exertion will vary for each person based on his or her level of fitness and previous experience with walking. My wife walks as her primary fitness tool, but it is not a Sunday stroll through the park. She can cover a mile walking faster than I can jogging! Now that may say something about the speed at which I run, but it illustrates that walking can be an aerobic experience!

The secret is to start slowly and build. Each week either increase the mileage or speed. When you have maxed out in those areas, look for more challenging terrain. A hill here and there can really spice up an otherwise tedious walk. Bring along a friend, your husband, or both! If you, like me, refer to this time as "my personal time" use it wisely for prayer or just clearing your head. You will be amazed at how many problems are unintentionally solved and how spiritual this time can be.

There are a few guidelines that will make your exercise routine more efficient and effective. First, throw away the pedometer and get a watch. Whether you are walking, running, doing aerobics, swimming, or rock climbing, it is the time involved and not the distance that matters. In other words, walk forty-five minutes instead of four miles. Studies show that it is the time not the mileage that burns fat and improves cardiovascular systems. If you are one of those who walks or runs at exactly the same pace at all times (hills and all), then the two measurements will be the same. In the real world, pace and effort can vary, so time spent in the activity is the most important factor in determining cardiovascular benefit.

If you want to increase the benefit, increase the time spent in the activity instead of the intensity. Increasing intensity or speed will burn fat quicker, but you still have to put in the time to get the maximum benefit. There is some recent research that reports the cardiovascular benefit of exercise can be obtained by doing brief stretches (ten minutes) of vigorous activity two to three times a day instead of a more continual program. This will certainly help the heart muscle, but it is not the most efficient way to burn fat. That is said with the understanding that you are already practicing the activity at a level that will do you some good. How do you know if you are? Your heartbeat should be elevated, and stay that way, in a range of 65 percent to 80 percent of its calculated maximum. (See table 13.)

Your breathing should be deep but not gasping for air, and again you should be able to carry on a conversation while exercising. Record your results. Keep a log of your activity and times. This will help you evaluate your progress and motivate you to continue.

I keep going back to aerobic exercise because of its overall benefit to all body systems. Here are a few common forms of exercise that, when done at the proper level of intensity, are aerobic: walking, running, bicycling, stationary biking, rowing, cross-country skiing, swimming, stair climbing, hiking, treadmill walking, roller skating, ice skating, in-line skating, class aerobics, bench aerobics, water aerobics, paying bills (just kidding).

What is surprising to people is the list of activities that are not usually aerobic. It doesn't mean these activities are not useful. Any movement is better than no movement. But the following activities

TABLE 13
CALCULATION OF MAXIMUM HEART RATE

220 minus age = maximum heart rate (applies if you don't have heart diseas or are on no medications that effect heart rate)

65 to 80 % of maximum heart rate = recommended training range

Example: 50-year-old woman with no heart disease, maximum heart rate would be 220-50 = 170
Recommended training heart rate would be 111–136

usually don't provide the continual heart rate elevation necessary to achieve aerobic benefit: tennis, golf, handball, racquetball, line dancing, softball, weightlifting, basketball, and sex (the intensity may be there, but usually not the duration). These provide excellent cross training or off day activities, but don't expect nine holes of golf three times a week to keep you fit and trim. Mix and match activities from both groups to avoid boredom and to keep your muscles fooled. An, ideal health program gets you doing something aerobic three days a minimum of thirty minutes, and then lets you do a nonaerobic activity on the alternate days.

REST

Don't forget about rest. Rest is an essential component of any exercise program. It is actually during the rest times that muscle is built and repaired. A fit person's body is burning more calories than that of a nonfit person, even at rest! You see, as you build your lean body mass (muscle), you increase the number of calories required to maintain that muscle. So even when you are sleeping, a fit person's body is burning more fuel to maintain and repair the often-used muscles.I was one of those obsessive exercisers until I learned this principle. I was continually developing minor injuries that were caused by nothing more than not allowing my body to rest and repair in between exercise.

Most of your won't have to worry about overtraining but keep in mind that rest is critical to continuing injury-free exercise. God knew the importance of rest. "On the seventh Day, Having fiinished his task, God rested from all his work"(Gen 2:2).

Thunder Thighs

Not long ago Millie came to me after a talk I gave and said."All this is about exercise is good and nice, and I even buy into the idea of it being good for me. But I want to know how to get rid of my thunder thighs and my cellulite."

First, I told her not to waste any money on rubs or creams, All those do is reduce the water content of the tissues and that will bounce right back. Second, I explained the reasons behind that ugly fat. In a woman this type of fat lies right under the skin and is called subcutaneuous fat. It is deposited first on the inside of the thigh, then on the outside of the thigh, Then the fat is placed on the hips, the middle, and then the upper body, mainly the area under the arms. This is a fact of female physiology, and it probably is a result of God's design to maximize the childbearing and nourishing ability of the female. How much goes to each area, and how quickly it gets there is genetically determined. (Thanks, Mom!) For the majority of women, these fat deposits are removed in the reverse order when fat is lost. In other words, as you begin fat-burning exercise the first deposits to come off are the upper body and arms followed by the middle and so on. The last bastion of fat is those thighs.

Spot reducing is a fantasy. It just doesn't happen. If you see someone who has just begun an exercise program and their hips and thighs are noticeably smaller, I would check their medical bills because it is likely they have paid a visit to their neighborhood plastic surgeon. To get rid of the thunder thighs and cellulite you must do aerobic exercise consistently and for whatever time it takes. For some it may be weeks; for others, months. There is no quick fix. Accept it, and get off your fanny and do something good for yourself. As my five-year-old loves to say, "Shake your boody."

Dr. George Sheehan, physician, author, and runner, said, "The choice is for fitness or fatness, to exercise or not to exercise. The ultimate cure for obesity is exercise."[2]

The main goals for exercise and fitness are to live better and prevent physical and emotional illness. Have you ever thought of exercise as a tool for healing? What about using exercise like you would a drug or a bandage? We are familiar with the use of exercise in the rehabilitation of heart attack patients. Everyone marvels at the physical therapy and devotion of the injured athlete striving to regain the competitive edge. What about the everyday aches and pains, the common ills that strike us? Can exercise be a healing influence? Sure it can. Let's look at how.

Aging

I think exercise is the fountain of youth. Dr. William Simpson, aging researcher and professor of Family Medicine at the Medical University of South Carolina states, "If we stay active many of the things that supposedly decline with age really don't decline."[3] Dr. Terrence Kavenaugh published a study of athletes, ages thirty-five to ninety-four, competing in the 1985 World Masters games and concluded, "These men and women were more typical of the average recreational sports person rather than the elite athlete. Yet the results of their exercise habits were marked. It seems that even modest exercise can push functional aging back 20 years."[4]

One of the biggest myths of aging is that older people don't need or benefit from exercise. Numerous studies point to just the opposite conclusion. The point is that light to moderate exercise, even in a ninety-year-old, can delay aging. More importantly it will improve the quality of life. A National Institute of Aging survey showed that only 27 percent of people over sixty-five exercise regularly. With those over sixty-five being the fastest-growing segment of the population today, it is critically important that these folks (and we will all be these folks sooner or later) be taught the benefits of exercise and be motivated to participate.

Will regular exercise help you live longer at a better quality of life? Yes, and once again science supports this. In a study of over 16,000 Harvard graduates followed over sixteen years, those who exercised moderately on a daily basis had a 33 percent lower death rate than their couch potato counterparts. My guess is that they had more fun also! A newsletter from the Baylor College of Medicine said, "The most exhausting part of exercising is the mental argument that takes place when you try to talk yourself into getting up off the couch and just doing it![5] Don't be like Barbara Johnson who said, "I have reached the point in life where the only thing I can exercise is caution!"[6]

Arthritis

Years ago doctors prescribed excessive rest for people struggling with osteoarthritis. The only problem with this regimen was that people consistently got worse rather than better. The approach to arthritis today is dramatically different. Studies over the past ten years have shown that simple exercise, such as walking and swimming, can be extremely therapeutic. Exercise can increase strength, flexibility, and, for some, allow them to cut back on their medications. Age and degree of arthritis doesn't appear to be a limiting factor. Dr. Donald Kay, who treats many arthritis patients said, "Even people in their mid-eighties have improved with exercise."[7]

The continued functioning of the joints, especially diseased joints, depends on their movement. Moving the joints increases the production of synovial fluid, the lubricant so essential in smooth joint operation. It also increases blood flow, which in turn reduces inflammation. Swimming has been identified as one of the best exercises for the woman bothered by arthritis, because of its low impact on the joints and its great range of motion capabilities. The growth of water aerobics programs around the country is testament to their effectiveness.

This is an area where you must develop an exercise program in concert with your doctor. There are rare types of bone and joint problems where exercise may not be as valuable, and you must have some parameters as far as intensity and type of exercise undertaken. See your doctor, jump in the pool, and put the Motrin on the shelf!

Constipation

I have yet to meet a woman who has had a baby who hasn't struggled with constipation (at some time in her life). Most people will experience this annoying problem occasionally, while some are afflicted on a regular or chronic basis. The secret to avoiding constipation is fiber, fluid, and fetch. We covered fiber and fluid in the chapter on diet. If you are not sure you are getting enough fiber or fluids, you probably aren't. Fetch stands for exercise, of course. (It was the only word starting with " f " I could come up with.)

Studies have actually looked at the transit time of food in the bowels and have discovered that people who exercise have a quicker rate of food passage. Many scientists believe that the faster transit time in exercisers is due to an increased secretion of hormones that stimulate bowel action. Sit ups, or any activity that increases the strength of the abdominal muscles, can enhance the passage of food in the intestines and can make its expulsion easier. Interestingly, Dr. Richard Miller, founder of the International Association of Yoga Therapists, claims that several of the twisting and turning motions of Yoga can enhance bowel motility. No studies to date are available, but the logic and anecdotal reports are interesting. An eighty-year-old lady gave me some advice several years back and I have never forgotten it. She said, "Honey, at my age, if my bowels are happy, I'm happy!"

Varicose Veins

I hate to disappoint you, but exercise will not get rid of the blue streak friends. What it can do is help prevent them from getting any worse, and, in some women, keep them from coming up at all. Varicosities are nothing more than dilated blood vessels. They arise secondary to the weakening of the vessel wall or due to stasis of the blood. Exercise gets the blood pumping, and forces the vessels to be more efficient at emptying. Some people may develop worse veins if they exercise and don't wear support hose, so check with your doctor. I had a patient who was twenty-four weeks pregnant and had the worst varicose veins I had ever encountered. They were actually painful, and the only way she was able to get relief was by running! The beneficial effect lasted for several hours after her run. She ran a mile the day before she went into labor!

Memory

Have you ever walked into a room and forgotten why you were there? Have you forgotten someone's name that you had known for twenty years? Research has shown that even these common memory lapses can be helped by regular exercise. A study done at Ohio State University took 72 people (average age of sixty-three) and had them ride stationary bikes three times a week for nine months. The researchers found that exercise improved attention span, concentration, and short-term memory.[8]

Robert Dustman, Ph.D., published a study from the VA hospital in Salt Lake City that showed a group of people between the ages of fifty-five and seventy could improve their memory and other cognitive measures by participating in a brisk walking program. He compared these patients with nonexercisers and a group that just used weights and did stretching. The walkers showed significant improvement over both groups.[9] Evidence shows that active people have a keener sense of visual recall. Some scientists have speculated that regular exercise increases the blood flow to the brain, and this may be responsible for the improved cognitive functioning.

Have you gotten the message yet? I think now you may better understand my admonition at the beginning of this chapter that exercise is not an option! There are unlimited types of activities that can be used for exercise from sitting in a chair lifting cans of soup to joining a local health club and becoming a gym rat. And there is always time. If you don't make time to exercise then you will have to make time to be sick.

ACTION CHALLENGE

1. Get a good physical exam.
2. Get started, today.
3. Do something aerobic, at least three times a week
4. Make it fun and something you enjoy.
5. Do it with a partner or group.
6. Be consistent and persistent.
7. Reap the benefits!

CHAPTER ELEVEN

Diet and Nutrition: Food for the Soul

How many times have you heard the old adage, "You are what you eat"? If you are like me, probably too many times. It is often spouted from the mouth of an anorexic-appearing aerobics queen who never had a weight problem in her life. Your first inclination is to waddle up to her and stuff wheat bran in her ear. But being the Christian woman that you are, you fight this temptation and smile and say, "Well, I guess that makes me a chocolate-covered Twinkie!"

The unfortunate thing about so many old adages is that many are true. And this is one of them. The fuel that we put in our bodies is the building block for every molecule, every organ, and every thought we have. The importance of food is illustrated by the obvious results of its deprivation. We die! Simple—end of story. I know that sounds trite and ridiculous, but I use that only to illustrate how important food is for normal functioning. We take it for granted. The good news is that healthy dietary habits can have a positive impact on your body and your soul.

SAD (Standard American Diet)

We are a nation of poor eaters. Some studies estimate that over 55 percent of the adult population can be categorized as obese. Fifteen percent to 40 percent of *children* are overweight. The nutritional habits that are formed in the early years influence us throughout our lives. Although you are past childhood, many of you have a child or teenager that respects your opinion (I realize including teenagers here is stretching reality), and you can have a major impact on their nutritional habits. The two most powerful teaching tools are the grocery cart and your example. You or your spouse buy the food that comes into the house. Granted, many kids eat at school and may have only one meal at home, but what that meal consists of and how it is prepared is your choice. This can't be a "Do as I say and not as I do" lesson. You must model good eating habits for those habits to have an impact on those around you.

Consider the health problems related to poor dietary practices. Heart disease, diabetes, stroke, cancer, and joint and bone problems are just a few of the maladies that are largely self-induced. Adhering to a few simple dietary guidelines can dramatically reduce the incidence of all these problems.

Normal Is Not Healthy

The standard American diet (SAD) that has been preached for years is fraught with myths, misperceptions, and downright lies. Over the next several pages I'll introduce some ideas about diet and nutrition that are biblically based and have special application to women in the midlife and menopause. I have already broached the subject of nutrition in the chapter on PMS, but I want to expand on some of those ideas and introduce you to some new ways of thinking about food.

When it comes to food you need to think abnormally! If you do what the "average American" does with her diet, then you will have the problems the average American has, namely clogged arteries, huge bellies, and thunder thighs. In this instance, normal is not healthy. If you strive to achieve the average daily allowances of calories and nutrients, the average intake of fats, carbohydrates, and proteins, and the average cholesterol, then you will probable have the average heart attack, the average stroke, or the average spare tire! Think abnormally; strive for what is truly healthy, not what is average. Don't fall into the trap of complacency by limiting yourself to "good enough" when it comes to your diet.

What The Bible Says

"Or don't you know that your body is the temple of the Holy Spirit, Who lives in you and was given to you by God? You do not belong to yourself, for God bought you with a high price. So you must honor God with your body." (1 Corinthians 6:19–20)

Paul, in his letter to the Corinthians, says that what you do with your body is important. You are not "free" to treat your body any way you please. That is a gross misinterpretation of free will. Your physical body, along with your spirit, belongs to God. The Life Application Bible commentary points out, "When we become Christians, the Holy Spirit comes to live in us. Therefore, we no longer own our bodies. That God bought us 'with a high price' refers to slaves purchased at an auction. Christ's death freed us from sin but also obligates us to His service. If you live in a building owned by someone else, you try not to violate the building's rules. Because your body belongs to God, you must not violate His standards for living. So many of the problems that we encounter in health and illness are due to not obeying the instructions of God."[1]

Granted there are many symptoms of the menopause and many illnesses of advanced age that are totally unrelated to diet and lifestyle; however, a quick survey of the leading causes of death in this country (heart disease and cancer) quickly shows that women are still doing something wrong.

Our longevity has dramatically improved, but much of that increase is due to the successful treatment of infectious diseases and improvement in public health and hygiene. We continue to have a major problem with "lifestyle" diseases such as heart disease, stroke, and some cancers. "Don't you realize that all of you together are the temple of God and that the Spirit of God lives in you? God will bring ruin upon anyone who ruins this temple. For God's temple is holy, and you Christians are that temple." (1 Cor. 3:16) Christians are called to glorify the temple (body) and it is obvious that the consequences of not doing so are great. You don't bring your trash to church, so don't feed trash to your body (temple).

Now the Good News

I don't want to paint a doom and gloom picture, because there is a great deal of good news on healthy living and healthy eating. Thankfully, it doesn't involve eating only kelp casseroles and cardboard! God didn't put you here without specific instructions on how to fuel this "temple of the Holy Spirit." That would be like giving you a new car but not telling you what it takes to make it go. You could try a great variety of different things, and you may eventually hit on the right fuel, but you will probably cause an excessive amount of damage before you find the right stuff. That is essentially what a lot of people do! They put all this garbage into their system and expect it to run like a Swiss watch. Wouldn't it make more sense for you to simply read the instructions? I admit that I am one of those people who opens the box and go at it before reading the "how to." I have a gadget graveyard to prove it. This is not smart or efficient. Almost any new device comes with that attention-getting warning on the first page of its manual: "IMPORTANT, read before using." New computer software comes with a "Read Me" file. The "Read Me" file for your internal computer is the Bible! So what does the Bible say about healthy eating?

A Holy Healthy Smorgasbord

God created specific substances for food. Just as He created man and woman for each other, so He created certain foodstuffs to be consumed. Look at Genesis chapter 1 verse 29–30: "And God said, `Look! I have given you the seed-bearing plants throughout the earth and all the fruit trees for your food. And I have given all the grasses and other green plants to the animals and birds for their food."

This is not too tough to figure out! God says that a predominately vegetarian diet is the healthiest. It is what He designed for us to use as fuels. These are the perfect foods! Anyone who is familiar with current nutritional research can tell you a diet based on fruits, vegetables, and plants is by far the most beneficial to one's health. Dr. Dean Ornish has become well known for his studies showing how a vegetarian diet can prevent heart disease. He has taken this a step further and has shown convincingly that the proper diet can actually reverse preexisting heart disease. Dr. Bob Arnot has a current bestseller that shows how a predominately vegetarian diet can actually reduce your risk of breast cancer.

None of These Diseases

I could go on and on about the scientific evidence supporting the health benefits of this approach, yet the best evidence lies in the pages of Scripture. Look at Exodus 15:25–26: "If you will listen carefully to the voice of the LORD your God and do what is right in His sight, obeying His commands and laws, then I will not make you suffer the diseases I sent on the Egyptians; for I am the LORD who heals you."

Notice that this promise is conditional. You must first *listen* to the instructions that God has given to you, and then you must *follow* them! If you do those two things then God has promised that you will not suffer any of the diseases of the Egyptians. What does this mean in today's world? You may be saying, "I don't have any Egyptian diseases, and don't plan on having any!"

If you look at the Egyptian culture at the time that Exodus was written, it is easy to understand the importance of this statement. The Egyptians of this era had begun to fundamentally change their diet from one which was grain-based to one which was meat-based. These were good and prosperous times. Meat was a luxury and a symbol of prosperity, so it was widely consumed by the wealthy during this era. As a result many Egyptians, especially the wealthy, developed the result of such a dietary shift... heart disease! Ancient writings are full of references to symptoms that are easily traced to atherosclerotic changes in blood vessels. The most compelling evidence is found in the well-preserved remains of mummies that actually show advanced atherosclerotic plaques in their arteries.

God says plainly that if you stick to the things that He created as food, then you will not suffer the diseases of those who choose foolishly. Remember that the first sin was not murder or adultery; it was eating something that God said man should not eat!

TABLE 14
HEALTHY FOODS OF THE BIBLE

Honey	Lentils
Nuts	Raisins
Fowl	Fruit
Figs	Barley
Beans	Spices
Herbs	Vegetables
Grapes	Cheese
Bread	Olives
Fish	Grain
Cucumbers	Vinegar
Melons	Garlic
Salt	Sheep

Adapted from *What the Bible Says about Healthy Living*

These verses establish "seed-bearing plants" as healthy food. This includes grains, beans, legumes, nuts, seeds, vegetables, fruits, herbs, and spices. (See Table 14.) The original variety of good foods is vast. If I stopped here, with a little imagination and creativity, you could create enough satisfying meals to last a lifetime.

However, God in His wisdom goes beyond this and adds to the smorgasbord. Look at Genesis 9:2–4: "All the wild animals, large and small, and all the birds and fish will be afraid of you. I have placed them in your power. I have given them to you for food, just as I have given you grain and vegetables. But you must never eat animals that still have their lifeblood in them."

God is giving instructions to Noah about how to live after the flood. It is important to understand that the eating of animals as described applied to "clean" animals. This designation was further explained in the Mosaic code in Deuteronomy 14:4–20.

> These are the animals you may eat: the ox, the sheep, the goat, the deer, the gazelle, the roebuck, the wild goat, the ibex, the antelope, and the mountain sheep.
>
> Any animal that has split hooves and chews the cud may be eaten, but if the animal doesn't have both, it may not be eaten. So you may not eat the camel, the hare, or the rock badger. They chew the cud but do not have split hooves. And the pig may not be eaten, for though it has split hooves, it does not chew the cud. All these animals are ceremonially unclean for you. You may not eat or even touch the dead bodies of such animals.
>
> As for marine animals, you may eat whatever has both fins and scales. You may not, however, eat marine animals that do not have both fins and scales. They are ceremonially unclean for you.
>
> You may eat any bird that is ceremonially clean. These are the birds you may not eat: the eagle, the vulture, the osprey, the buzzard, kites of all kinds, ravens of all kinds, the ostrich, the nighthawk, the seagull, hawks of all kinds, the little owl, the great owl, the white owl, the pelican, the carrion vulture, the cormorant, the stork, herons of all kinds, the hoopoe, and the bat.All flying insects are ceremonially unclean for you and may not be eaten. But you may eat any winged creature that is ceremonially clean.

In Genesis, when God is talking about grains and seed-bearing plants, the translations are consistent in saying you shall eat these substances. This is in the form of a command, a directive. Yet in Deuteronomy, when referring to the use of animals as food, the wording is distinctly different. As Dr. Rex Russell observes, time and time again the term *may* is used. This is done for a reason. God intended the use of seed bearing plants and fruits as the foundation for healthy diets. However, He allows us to choose certain meats to supplement our diet. Under no circumstances was it to be implied that meats and animals were to be the basic building blocks for our nutrition.

Clean and Unclean

By examining further this important distinction between clean and unclean meats, we see that God states it is permissible to eat "clean" animals and totally wrong to consume the "unclean." What is the difference?

In today's language it would be a normal and simplistic assumption to believe that God was commanding man to stay away from dirty food. That may be true, but that is not the correct interpretation of the terms. According to scholars, a clean animal is defined by what it eats and the cleanliness of its digestive tract.

If you refer back to the laws in Deuteronomy, the only clean animals are those that have divided hooves and chew the cud. It is no surprise that the only animals that fit both categories are the animals that consume vegetarian diets themselves! The scavengers and the flesh eaters are considered unclean. (See Table 15 for a list of clean and unclean animals.) By avoiding those animals that consumed other animals, people avoided many of the diseases that were transmitted by the likes of parasites and worms. The group of unclean animals is called omnivores, because they literally will eat anything. What they eat in turn will be reflected in what you eat. This prohibition from consuming unclean animals protected the Israelites from many of the diseases that were transmitted by means of bacteria and parasites.

Does this distinction apply in today's world of strict manufacturing standards and quality control? Absolutely! The benefit in excluding the "unclean" animals today is not derived from the

TABLE 15
CLEAN AND UNCLEAN ANIMALS

Clean Animals	Unclean Animals
Calf	Clams
Deer	Catfish
Goat	Shrimp
Ox	Pigs
Sheep	Rabbit
Chicken	Ostrich
Duck	Squirrel
Turkey	Crabs
Cod	Oyster
Flounder	Opossum
Halibut	Lobster
Salmon	Tuna

standpoint of communicable disease, but from the avoidance of the consequences of high saturated fat, low fiber diets.

God has a design, and the charge is to abide by it. Remember you are "fearfully and wonderfully made," but you are also responsible to honor God's instructions.

It is important to also understand the distinction between clean and unclean in describing one's spirituality. Abiding by these dietary laws does not imply any greater degree of spiritual attainment; all they refer to is the physical well-being of those who practice these habits. So don't confuse the issues with the terminology. You don't achieve spiritual cleanliness by keeping certain dietary restrictions. Old Testament dietary laws are not a way to earn entry into the kingdom of heaven, but they are a way to keep us healthy along the path.

Paul (in 1 Corinthians and Galatians) Paul says eating clean or unclean animals does not have any spiritual value itself However, God has given us a plan that if followed will provide us with optimal health. The reason to follow these instructions is to glorify God by acknowledging His desire and design for our health.

FAT IS NOT WHERE IT IS AT

Excessive fat intake is associated with a multitude of health problems. Atherosclerotic heart disease, the leading killer of adults, is intimately linked to dietary fat intake. High LDL cholesterol, diabetes, stroke, and obesity are all increased by a diet high in saturated fats. It is common knowledge that the leading source of saturated fats in the average diet is from meat and meat products. The logic is clear. If you reduce the intake of bad fats, you will inevitably reduce the likelihood of developing this myriad of debilitating diseases.

Some fat is good, in fact necessary, for proper body functioning. The key is moderating your intake and being careful of the type of fat. It has never been easier to quantify fat intake. Virtually every food product packaged and sold has nutritional labels that clearly state the fat content and its corresponding components. Saturated fat is the bad guy. That is what helps clog the pipes.

What I find interesting is that some people think this is a new finding. The fallacy is that only through the miracle of modern science and the high-tech advances in testing have we been able to come to these conclusions. Imagine my surprise when I found Leviticus 7:23–27: "Give the Israelites these instructions: You must never eat fat, whether from oxen or sheep or goats. The fat of an animal found dead or killed by a wild animal may never be eaten, though it may be used for any other purpose. Anyone who eats fat from an offering given to the LORD by fire must be cut off from the community. Even in your homes, you must never eat the blood of any bird or animal. Anyone who eats blood must be cut off from the community."

Dr. Rex Russell summarizes a healthy approach to fat consumption in his marvelous book *What the Bible Says about Healthy Living*. "Enjoy any fat found in a created foodnuts, seeds, fruits, vegetables, and legumes. We can enjoy pure butter and any unrefined liquid oils that have been protected from air, light, heat, and chemicals. They have proven to be better for us than chemically extracted oils. The best oils for cooking are virgin olive oil and butter. Even fat found in the marbled flesh of "clean" animals, birds, or fish is healthful." What should be avoided? Processed oils, hormone or antibiotic laden animals, cover fat or suet, margarine, and meat eating animals.[2]

God, the Great Designer, knew what was best for His creation long before the invention of cholesterol measuring devices or cardiac stress tests!

The Horn of Plenty

Christianity is a religion of abundance. We believe in a gracious and loving God. It follows that God doesn't spend all His time telling folks what not to eat. He also makes it clear what is good fuel for our bodies. As we have already seen in Genesis 1:29, God gave us the seed bearing plants and fruit trees. The Bible also mentions several other foods as being healthy and wholesome. For example, Ezekiel 16:8 gives the secret to beauty: "You ate the finest foods-fine flour, honey, and olive oil-and became more beautiful than ever." I am not advocating a crash diet of honey and olive oil to get rid of cellulite and wrinkles, but any knowledgeable nutritionist touts the health benefits of these substances, especially when they are used instead of their synthetic, processed counterparts.

The Old Testament does not hold a monopoly on healthy nutrition. The writers of the Gospels were also inspired to give instructions for healthy dietary intake. They make specific points of referencing certain foods eaten by Jesus and his followers. I don't think it is by accident that these foods are specifically mentioned. Look at Matthew 15:36: "Then he took the seven loaves and the fish, thanked God for them, broke them into pieces, and gave them to the disciples, who distributed the food to the crowd." He didn't feed the five thousand with steak and eggs! Now granted, bread and fish were the staples of the people in Judea in the first century. However, the significance of this miracle is not just in the feeding of the masses, but also with the foodstuffs with which it was done.

AMOUNTS COUNT

There is a tremendous variety and selection of food available that has been literally blessed by God. These foods are abundant, and when used properly, will provide the cornerstone of any healthy lifestyle. A word of caution about overdoing it: We have already alluded to the tremendous problems associated with obesity. Some estimates say over 50 percent of the adult population is overweight. Based on my observations, that is a conservative estimate! The point is that you can get fat by eating only the "right" foods. Let me say it again. You can become large, heavy, "big boned," and blimpish from eating *too much* of the good stuff.

God set the guidelines many years ago in Deuteronomy 32:15, "But Israel soon became fat and unruly; the people grew heavy, plump, and stuffed! Then they abandoned the God who had made them." Proverbs 23:1 reinforces this point: "When dining with a ruler, pay attention to what is put before you. If you are a big eater put a knife to your throat, and don't desire all the delicacies–deception may be involved." Some may consider attempting to cut your throat a bit drastic in the battle against the bulge, but this only reinforces how moderation and discipline pave the way to dietary success. There is no health benefit in being heavy, plump, and stuffed! Keep all things in moderation, even the good stuff!

Another implied concept from Jewish dietary laws is that food was largely consumed in its natural, raw, uncooked state in centuries past. There is no evidence in Scripture that says directly that cooking food is bad. Common sense says that, especially when it comes to meat, cooking is a preferable method of preparation (my apologies to the sushi lovers). However, fruits, grains, vegetables, and seeds should be consumed in their natural state. We know that many of the problems associated with diets are not so much the foods themselves but the method of preparation. Lose the grease, put out the fire, and eat it raw! Luckily there are many more resources for organically grown vegetables today than there were in the past. It's more inconvenient, and often more expensive, yet the long term benefits are undeniable.

Many foods play a significant role in minimizing specific problems associated with the menopause. Soy and soy products contain phytoestrogens, or substances with estrogen-like activity, which can be effective in attacking symptoms alone or in combination with other therapies. Foods such as leafy green vegetables and sea plants contain a great deal of calcium, which is critical in the menopausal years. I will spend a great deal of time discussing these specific dietary habits in the chapter on menopause. These dietary instructions apply not only to midlife but from cradle to grave.

SUMMARY

You are what you eat. God has said that a diet based largely on vegetables, fruits, and plants is healthy and fights disease. The midlife and menopause is a time for change, and one positive change is to shift your diet to one that will not only reduce menopausal symptoms but also improve your overall state of health. Some "clean" meats are acceptable, but everything should be weighed in the scale of moderation. The admonition, "Teach your children well," certainly applies to your responsibility to instruct those that respect and depend on you for advice about foods. Think abnormally! Strive to be unaverage in what you eat and how much of it you eat.

ACTION CHALLENGE

Write down everything you eat, morning, noon, and night, for a week. Read the list at the week's end and. Then after a good cry, identify' areas of weakness. Do you tend to overdo it more at night or in the morning? Are McDonald's lunches your downfall? This can be an enlightening (and frightening) exercise, yet it is the foundation for initiating healthy change.

CHAPTER TWELVE

Osteoporosis: Dem Bones

Osteoporosis has the potential to be one of the most important words in your health vocabulary. The next time you are in church (you know you should be), look to your immediate left and look to your immediate right. You will see women severely affected by osteoporosis. I want to be sure you understand the definitions and terms before we spend too much time on the grim statistics.

Osteoporosis means "porous bone." Call it brittle bones or thinning bones; it all means the same thing. The technical definition is a skeletal disease characterized by low bone mass and microarchitectural deterioration of bone tissue, leading to enhanced bone fragility and a consequent increase in fracture risk. The plain English translation is a thinning of the material that makes the bones strong that may result in an increased risk for bone breaks. Osteoporosis is a disease, a preventable disease. Osteoporosis can be identified early, and measures can be taken to slow or stop its progression. The goal is to prevent the clinical result of the disease, fractures. Understand-no one ever died of osteoporosis. What women die from are complications of the disease, that is, the fractures and their subsequent results.

Today's technology can now detect osteoporosis in its early stages, and this allows for aggressive and successful treatments. In addition, we now know who is at increased risk for developing osteoporosis. With this knowledge, these high-risk women can take steps to make sure they are not one of the 250,000 who will suffer osteoporotic-related fractures next year.

Bones Are Alive

The bone is a living, dynamic tissue. It is constantly being constructed and broken down. The trabecular bone is the site for the majority of this activity. This is the internal part of the bone that

Table 16
Clinical Types of Osteoporosis

Primary	
Postmenopausal	
Aging (men and women)	
Secondary	
Renal failure	Hyperthyroidism
Intestinal bypass	Cushings syndrome
Malabsorption syndromes	Rheumatoid arthritis
Multiple myeloma	Anticonvulsants
Cancer	Antacids (chronic abuse)
Diabetes	Thyroid hormone therapy

gives it most of its strength and stability. When more bone is being broken down than is being built up the net result is a weaker, less stable bone. Women are far more likely to be affected than men, especially after the menopause. This is due in part to estrogen's effect on the osteoblast (bone-building cells) and osteoclast (bone-eating cells). Estrogen stimulates the osteoblast (bone-building) and blocks the osteoclast (bone-eating). This serves to protect the female while significant amounts of estrogen are circulating in her bloodstream. After the menopause, when estrogen levels decline, the osteoblast are not as aggressive in building bone and the osteoclast are hungrier and eat up more bone. The net result is an acceleration of bone loss at menopause. This is significant because it is this loss of the trabecular bone in the hip and leg that leads to the increased risk for fractures a few years down the road.

There are many other factors that control bone loss, but for the sake of our discussion, and the fact that these other causes are relatively rare, I will limit this discussion to estrogen-deficiency-related osteoporosis. I have listed some of the other causes in Table 16.

Again, osteoporosis is the condition, and a fracture is a complication of the condition. You want to do everything you can to avoid developing osteoporosis, which in turn prevents pathological fractures.

Scare Tactics

Should you be concerned about osteoporosis? Consider the statistics. Over 250,000 women every year suffer a hip fracture directly or indirectly related to osteoporosis. If this number isn't frightening by itself, the long-term results of hip fractures are alarming. Up to 20 percent of women who fracture their hip die in the year after the break due to complications of the fracture. Of those who survive, almost 50 percent end up in a nursing home or an extended care facility. Twenty-five million women are affected by osteoporosis. The medical economists estimate that hip fractures alone account for upwards of 10 billion dollars a year in health care costs. Nearly 33 percent of women will fracture their hips in their lifetimes, and the greatest single risk factor is osteoporosis. But remember, the good news is that this is a preventable disease!

The women at greatest risk of developing osteoporosis are thin, Caucasian, and inactive. In talks I tell audiences that the little old white lady who has Twinkies and Jack Daniels for breakfast, cigarettes for lunch, and watches soap operas all day will definitely have brittle bones (among other things). See Table 17 for a listing of the common risk factors for osteoporosis. Not everyone develops osteoporosis. But as you can see, women in the menopausal age group have a greater likelihood of doing so.

Any woman over the age of fifty automatically falls into a high-risk category. Look at the list closely and identify how many risk factors you have. Notice that only a select few are unalterable, such as family history. (It really is a shame we can't pick our parents!)

TABLE 17
RISK FACTORS FOR OSTEOPOROSIS

Caucasian
Oriental
Early menopause
Turner's syndrome
Small, thin frame
Poor diet
Caffeine intake
High protein diet
Smoking
Physical inactivity
Alcohol
Late puberty
Prior hysterectomy
Few or infrequent periods
Eating disorders (anorexia, bulemia)
Scoliosis
Family history

The point is that the vast majority of characteristics that put you in a high-risk category are behaviors and choices that you control. The writer of Proverbs knew this when he wrote, "A merry heart does good, like medicine, but a broken spirit dries the bones." Solomon also says in Proverbs 3:7–8, "Do not be wise in your own eyes; fear the Lord and depart from evil. It will be health to your flesh, and strength to your bones."

What To Do?

The prevention of osteoporosis should be the next great success story of public health education. The four A's pave the road to osteoporosis prevention.

Attitude: Take a proactive role in making decisions to alter behavior and lifestyle. Look again at the risk factors. What are the changes you can make beginning tomorrow that will minimize your potential for bone loss? Don't fall into the trap of procrastination. Studies are conclusive in showing that the earlier in life these healthy decisions are made, the less likely it is there will be trouble later on. The biggest obstacle I have found in osteoporosis attitude adjustment is that people are not motivated to change. They feel fine. They don't have any outward or inward sign that this process is progressing. It's not like gaining weight, where the results are all too obvious. People have no forewarning before it is late in the game.The truth is that now we have ways of detecting these changes very early but the technology is still underutilized. (More about this later.) The ideal situation is to never need the technology. Change your attitude from the "head in the sand" mentality to one of prevention. "The light of the eyes rejoices the heart, and a good report makes the bones healthy" (Prov. 15:30).

Aptitude: Learn everything you can concerning methods to prevent osteoporosis. Many women don't make the necessary lifestyle changes because they simply aren't aware of what changes to make! They don't know what behaviors make them more susceptible to bone loss. It's hard to be preventive when you don't know where to start. Next, learn all you can about different approaches to prevention including medications, diet, and exercise. Read on and you will fulfill this objective.

Action: Here we go again! Exercise, exercise, and more exercise. Weight-bearing exercise is a vital tool in preventing bone loss. Every study that has evaluated the relationship between exercise and osteoporosis has shown a strong protective effect. Weight-bearing exercise strengthens bone and reduces its breakdown. This includes running, aerobic exercising, weightlifting, dancing, using treadmills, ski machines, and anything that puts strain on the bones. Swimming doesn't seem to provide much benefit because the water supports the bones. When bone has pressure applied to it through weight-bearing exercise, over an extended period of time, its density will increase. The pressure applied from muscle contractions, gravity, and the demands of exercise actually stimulates calcium deposition in the bone structure. The best thing a woman can do to strengthen her bones is to get active.

Apothecary: There are several medications, herbs, foods and vitamins that are important in the osteoporosis story. First, let's talk about diet.

Certain dietary excesses and deficiencies have been associated with increased bone loss. Luckily these are fairly rare for the average woman. Prevention can be as much about avoidance of bad things as it is consuming the right things. Unusual dietary habits that may promote osteoporosis include low calcium intake, high phosphorous intake, high-protein diets (a common weight-loss approach), excessive salt intake, and high sugar diets. All of these approaches can, over time, increase the metabolic loss of bone. This is not a rapid effect, so a week of high protein intake will not cause osteoporosis, but consistently eating excessive amounts of protein can increase the leeching of calcium from the bone leading to bone structure deterioration.

What is the highest source of phosphates in the average diet? Soft drinks! The woman who drinks a six-pack of diet cola a day (and you would be amazed how many do) is increasing her risk for brittle bones in the future. This will really have an impact as the baby boomers age since they are the first generation that has consumed soft drinks in mass quantities from an early age. Remember bone loss is cumulative, so the more you lose early on, the greater your risk later in life.

Do The Right Thing

Enough of the negative. Let's focus on the proactive things a woman can embrace to reduce or possibly prevent osteoporosis. A vegetarian diet is associated with a lower risk of osteoporosis. Marsh and colleagues showed this in their paper comparing lactovegetarians and omnivores published in the *American Journal of Clinical Nutrition* in 1983.[1] This may be due, they speculate, to the decreased protein intake in a vegetarian diet."

"And God said, 'Look! I have given you the seed-bearing plants throughout the earth and all the fruit trees for your food'." It is no surprise that God's food gifts were the same that would optimally maintain His creation. Green leafy vegetables are the major components of a vegetarian diet that aid in preventing bone loss. They serve as an important source of boron, calcium, and vitamin K. Vitamin K is essential to the proper mineralization of the bone, and deficiencies can increase the severity of bone fractures. Boron is an essential ingredient in the proper interaction of vitamin D and estrogen on the bone. The consumption of phytoestrogens (see chapter on diet) may help in the overall battle against osteoporosis. Some of the isoflavonoids in plants are being investigated for their interaction with calcitonin, a hormone that regulates calcium metabolism.

Calcium tends to get the headlines, but several other vitamins and minerals are also important in proper bone health. Vitamin D helps to regulate how the kidneys excrete calcium. This in turn controls the blood level of calcium, which directly impacts the absorption rate from the bone. Vitamin D deficiency can be manifested in the older population who may not get much sun exposure (sun causes a chemical change in the skin that forms vitamin D). Studies support the recommendation to consume at least 400 IU of vitamin D a day, either through diet or supplements. I have yet to see a good and accurate measure of vitamin D content in specific foods, so I have found it much easier to make sure I am getting enough by taking a supplement.

Magnesium is the mineral that gets no respect. When it comes to osteoporosis, calcium and vitamins get all the press, but magnesium is very important. Magnesium activates enzymes that help form new calcium crystals. It is also important in helping vitamin D convert to its active form, and in helping with proper function of the bone-related hormones: parathyroid hormone and calcitonin.

Women with severe osteoporosis have a lower magnesium level in their blood than women without osteoporosis.[2] A 1990 study looked at combining adequate calcium with magnesium and found this regimen not only decreased bone loss, but also increased the remineralization of weight bearing bones.[3] Ingesting the proper ratio of magnesium and calcium is more effective than simply taking calcium. Research has suggested that the optimal magnesium intake is 400-800 mg per day.

Manganese, folic acid, strontium, vitamin B6, vitamin B12, and silicon have all been linked to good bone health. Most are critical components in the bone formation process, and without their proper concentration this formation of bone does not proceed with maximal efficiency. In reality, a good diet will provide plenty of each of these vitamins and minerals, so specific supplementation is not needed. Most good multivitamin formulations will contain adequate amounts of all of these.

Calcium

Calcium is well-known as the critical mineral in osteoporosis prevention. There is no question that calcium supplementation has been shown to reduce bone loss in postmenopausal women.[4] More importantly, calcium added to the diet has been shown to reduce the incidence of the dreaded consequence of osteoporosis, the fracture. Calcium is a major component of trabecular bone matrix, and without adequate amounts of calcium, the proper bone consistency cannot be maintained.

Over the years there has been a lot of debate about the proper amount and form of calcium to utilize. The National Institute of Health and the National Academy of Sciences recommend 1,000-1,200 mg of calcium a day for women under sixty-five and 1,500 mg a day for those over sixty-five. These recommendations are based on years of research and data.[5] These are total daily dietary intake amounts. The reality is that most standard American diets only provide about 500-800 mg of calcium a day. For those who don't consume dairy products or many vegetables, this value may be even less.

It follows then, that to get adequate calcium without a major change in diet you must supplement. Based on the data, a supplement with at least 500 mg of calcium is recommended.

Calcium carbonate is one of the most readily available calcium supplements. It is the form of calcium in products such as Tums EX, Os-cal, and Caltrate. Some argue that calcium citrate is better absorbed; yet research suggests that the true clinical value of this increased absorption is negligible. I have found that the most important factor is tolerability. Some calcium products irritate the gastrointestinal tract causing stomach upset or diarrhea. This problem is individualized and may even vary from product to product. Trial and error is the best method to determine which calcium supplement is right for you.

Another advantage of refined calcium carbonate is its low lead content. Calcium derived from oyster shells, dolomite, or bone meal may contain undesirable amounts of lead that could negatively impact your health if taken over a long period of time. Other good sources of calcium are those combined with citrate, gluconate, or fumerate. Read the labels. It will say specifically on the label what type of calcium it contains and the amount.

Parade of Stars

Five medications have an impact on osteoporosis: estrogen, progesterone, alendronate, raloxifene, and calcitonin.

The studies are voluminous and conclusive that taking estrogen reduces bone loss. Even the most radical critics agree that estrogen loss at menopause accelerates overall bone loss, and the use of estrogen can slow the process.[6] Is estrogen use the only way to prevent osteoporosis? Will you become a hump-backed, creaky old lady if you don't use estrogen (as some of the drug companies subtly imply)? Absolutely not!

There are options. Can estrogen be an important part of osteoporosis prevention and treatment? You bet it can! It is all about balance. Are you at high risk for osteoporosis? Are you doing the right things with your diet and exercise? Can the advantages of

HRT override the risks for your individual situation? These are the kind of questions that must be answered when considering a medication like estrogen. For many, this is most efficiently done in consultation with a health care provider that is well-versed on options. Be sure they are knowledgeable on all alternatives. How do you know if they are? Ask!

With this book as a foundation, you can ask them about diet, herbs, vitamins and other medications. Remember to explore your options. If you do choose to go with HRT, consider estradiol (E2). The Tri-est formulation has not been tested enough over time to be shown effective in preventing fractures. Logically, one would assume it would be so, but the data is just not there yet.

The role of progesterone in bone physiology is not clear. There are progesterone receptors on the osteoblast (bone-builders), yet the exact effect of progesterone on these cells has not been determined. In laboratory experiments progesterone has been shown to promote bone growth in animals, but this has not convincingly been shown in humans. In women who have a known progesterone deficiency (anovulatory), there is a measurable increase in the rate of bone loss when compared to those women with normal blood progesterone levels. This provides presumptive evidence that progesterone is linked to bone metabolism. What is lacking is a long-term study of natural progesterone replacement (comparing bone loss or gain to a placebo) and then a follow-up of these patients for several years to see if there is an actual decrease in the fracture incidence. There is some data that suggests the addition of natural progesterone to estrogen regimens enhances the overall bone sparing ability.

Dr. John Lee, in his book *What Your Doctor May Not Tell You about Menopause*, claims that natural progesterone cream not only slows bone loss but also actually builds bone. This is premature, and the data just doesn't support using progesterone <u>cream</u> as a way to prevent bone loss. Even some of his data is from women on both estrogen and progesterone. Several of the studies he quotes to support his arguments are from work done on micronized progesterone, an oral form that differs in absorption from the cream. These studies had very small numbers of participants, and it is invalid to take those results and assume the same would apply for the cream.

Dr. Jerilynn Prior of the University of British Columbia has done a great deal of research on bone and menstrual cycle irregularity in athletes. Lee and others often quote her as a source of evidence for the use of progesterone in osteoporosis prevention. However, her work, if you actually read the studies, is on a very specific population and is largely observational. Natural progesterone cream has not been tested as to its long-term effect on osteoporosis by her or any one else that I could find in a recent literature search. The take-home message is that natural progesterone cream has many useful applications; however, using it as your sole aid against osteoporosis is wrong and dangerous.

Alendronate (Fosamax) is a drug known as a biphosphanate that is approved by the FDA for the prevention and treatment of postmenopausal osteoporosis. It works directly on the bone to prevent bone breakdown by blocking the action of the osteoclasts (boneeaters). Its only benefit is on the bone, and it will do nothing to counteract any of the other symptoms of menopause. Alendronate's long-term safety has yet to be determined, although short-term safety has been well tested.

The biggest problem with Alendronate is how it is dosed. To get proper absorption, it must be swallowed on an empty stomach, and then the woman must remain upright and without food for thirty minutes. It doesn't sound complicated, but in my practice it has proven to be a deterrent to compliance. Anything that interferes with convenience lessens compliance. I have also seen patients complain of digestive discomfort and esophagitis (reflux). There is no doubt that the medicine is effective at reducing bone loss. Once again, it becomes an individual decision as to whether the advantages outweigh the disadvantages for your situation.

Calcitonin is a hormone produced by the thyroid gland that is responsible for calcium use in the bone. It is approved by the FDA for treatment, not prevention, of osteoporosis. It should only be considered in patients with already diagnosed osteoporosis. It actually increases bone density and may reduce bone pain from fractures and osteoporotic changes. It is given by injection or a nasal spray. In the short term it is a safe medication, but again the long-term studies of safety are lacking.

Raloxifene (Evista) is one of a new class of medications called the SERMs. This stands for selective estrogen receptor modulators. They have been nicknamed "designer estrogens" by the media. What that means in real English is that these drugs selectively attach to certain receptors and avoid other similar receptors. In the case of Raloxifene, it stimulates the estrogen receptors in the bone but not in the uterus. In the breast it actually appears to act as an anti-estrogen. In fact, when this drug was first being tested it was being evaluated as a possible treatment for breast cancer. The beneficial effects on bone were first noted as a welcomed side effect; however, as the research developed, it was found that the bone benefit was truly remarkable and marketable. Even though it is a hormone with some estrogen-like effects, it will not counteract any of the other menopausal symptoms. In fact, a number of women using Raloxifene will experience hot flashes. Women with a uterus can use this safely, as there is no effect or increased risk for uterine overgrowth, bleeding, or cancer.

At the time of this writing researchers have been following patients on Raloxifene for forty months and have seen a 40 per reduction in the occurrence of breast cancer as compared to the general population. This data is preliminary but encouraging. Women may soon have a medication that will help osteoporosis and possibly reduce the incidence of breast cancer. It is still too early to make that claim, however. Another potential benefit of Raloxifene is that there appears to be a lowering of total cholesterol in users as compared to the general population. Whether this will have a clinical effect on the reduction of heart disease remains to be seen.

Medications, Who Needs Them?

Who should consider using these medications? Anyone who is in a high-risk position! And that means about all women in the menopause. Hear what I said: *Consider* using something. Look at your options. Should everyone use these medications? Absolutely not! Anyone who suggests that all women over the age of fifty should be on medication is wrong. These medicines are only to be considered after making the proper lifestyle changes, dietary modifications, and exercise. I see many women who want the easy way out. They want to take a pill and continue to smoke, be lazy, and eat garbage. This is dangerous and detrimental to their health. Health is balance, and this approach is anything but healthy.

I mentioned earlier that the technology exists to identify osteoporosis in its early stages. This is known as bone densiometry. You may hear of it as BMD or bone mineral densiometry. This technique uses x-ray technology and computer calculations to assess the density or mass of individual bones or the entire body. The gold standard in BMD measurement is the DEXA, or dual-energy x-ray absorptiometry, because of its precision and accuracy. The most common areas tested are the lumbar spine and the hip, mainly because these are the two areas most profoundly affected by osteoporosis.

The National Osteoporosis Foundation has published guidelines as to who should have BMD measurements. These are found in Table 18.

In general, anyone who is considering using a medication to prevent osteoporosis, has a strong family history of the disease, or has two or more high risk factors should get a bone densiometry. Universal screening is not needed, and whether or not a person gets a bone densiometry is dependent on her own medical situation and her risk factors.

Other cheaper and simpler methods of detecting bone loss are available; however, they suffer from the lack of accuracy and specificity. The heel ultrasound is a small office-based machine that measures differences in bone reflection of sound waves and has been shown to be accurate in predicting fracture risk. It is a screening device in that an abnormal result needs to be followed by a regular BMD to determine if osteoporosis is present and the anatomical location where it is most likely to be a problem. Ultrasound is easy to do, painless, and inexpensive, so it functions well as a first approach

TABLE 18
BONE DENSIOMETRY GUIDELINES

- All postmenopausal women under 65 who have one or more additional risk factors
- All women 65 and over
- Postmenopausal women who present with fractures
- Women who are considering therapy for osteoporosis, if BMD would facilitate the decision
- Women who have been on hormone replacement therapy for prolonged periods

to screening the right individuals. It is less sensitive, so it should only be done every couple of years to give meaningful serial data.

Two other bone-related tests you should be familiar with are measures of bone loss and bone formation. These are most useful in following the effectiveness of therapy. They cannot be used by themselves to make a diagnosis of osteoporosis. If someone is taking a medication and is curious about whether it is working or not, they can opt for one of these approaches. The bone-loss test checks the urine for bone breakdown products while the bone-buildup evaluation is a blood test that looks at the byproduct of bone production. Both are fairly accurate. They can be useful in assessing whether a certain regimen is working, and may contribute to the decision to continue your present treatment or change directions.

ACTION CHALLENGE

Prevention

1. Identify and minimize risk factors.
2. Consider bone densiometry.
3. Eat a vegetarian-based diet.

4. Exercise (weight-bearing).
5. Get adequate calcium (500-800 mg/day), magnesium (400-800 mg/day), boron (3-5 mg/day).
6. Consider HRT or Raloxifene if high-risk.
7. Follow effectiveness with urine or blood tests.

Treatment

1. Have a DEXA bone mineral density test.
2. Take HRT, Alendronate, Raloxifene, or Calcitonin.
3. Follow all the prevention suggestions.

CHAPTER THIRTEEN

The Healing Power of Prayer

Prayer heals! Whether it is PMS, menopause, AIDS, or cancer, I believe strongly that your physical health and mental well-being are intimately linked to your spiritual health. This is not meant to imply that the only way to physical health is through religion. Don't misunderstand. There are many physically and mentally healthy individuals who have no interest in their spiritual side. However, to achieve joyous well-being and balance, the soul can't be excluded. Daily prayer can be as vital to a healthy midlife experience as exercise, herbs, and diet. I challenge you to open your mind and heart to the possibility that prayer can be a powerful mode of healing and an essential part of health. I see prayer as the thread that is woven throughout the tapestry of midlife giving it strength and unity.

For many, the association of prayer and healing is a natural one. It is easy to put the two together. For others, the idea of prayer and healing may be a stretch. The only identification some see with prayer and healing is a self-righteous TV evangelist laying on hands and yelling, "Be gone, you evil hot-flash demon!" That is not the type of healing prayer that I am concerned with.

Prayer as a Daily Tool

Think about using prayer as a daily tool for healthy living. Just as you would get up in the morning and brush your teeth (or soak your dentures) and reach for the vitamins, so you could (and should) have prayer as a part of your daily regimen. For a long time I, like many others, thought of prayer in a last-resort mentality: When all else fails, try prayer. Prayer is the only thing that will help now.

I lived under this falsehood for the first few years of my practice. I would pray for folks when nothing else I, or any other doctor, could do would alter the outcome. Through prayer and study, but mostly through my patients, I leamed that this is only a superficial utilization of prayer. It's like giving a fraction of the proper dose of penicillin and hoping it kills the germ. The reality is that I had a full dose of antibiotic just waiting to be injected. So it is with prayer. Don't wait until you are sick to utilize this wonderful and powerful gift.

I want to stimulate you to begin to see prayer as a vital, daily part of your quest for health. In addition I want to show you some of the scientific evidence that supports the healing power of prayer.

Three Models of Healing

A while ago, my younger brother Bruce went in the hospital for emergency surgery to remove his severely infected appendix. As I was thinking about him, it occurred to me that during his hospitalization and recovery he would deal with three distinct yet interrelated modes of healing.

The first, and by far the most immediate, is the mechanical mode of healing. This is surgery to remove the infected tissue. No intelligent person would disagree that this is a necessary and helpful tool in this situation. Before surgery and anesthesia was made safe, many died from rupture of the appendix and subsequent sepsis. So utilizing the mechanical healing model is highly effective and desirable in this scenario.

The second mode of healing that is available to Bruce is mind-body healing, the mental mode. This is healing that is influenced by how we think, feel, and believe. Unfortunately many Christians have incorrectly associated this type of healing with New Age philosophies, so they have a barrier to overcome before accepting the legitimacy of this healing tool. God designed this relationship between mind and body as part of His perfect plan for our healthy existence. We are much more than just our physical bodies.

How we feel about an illness can dramatically affect its course. There is a new branch of science called psychoneuroimmunology that studies how thoughts and emotions impact our immune system. It has been scientifically proven that emotions such as anxiety and anger can actually decrease the function of white blood cells, our body's defense against disease. So, how stressed Bruce is, how much faith he has in his surgeon, and his belief about his own state of health all can impact his healing.

The third mode of healing that I envision for Bruce is the healing power of prayer, the spiritual mode. To date this has not been as scientifically studied as the first two modes, yet I firmly believe its role is just as powerful and effective as the other two. In fact, it predates the other two as a healing tool. Prayer has long been associated with healing, and it is only recently that this unnatural separation has developed.

These three approaches are not exclusive to one another. They work best to achieve healing when they work together. The wise person is the one who doesn't focus on only one tool but embraces all the gifts of grace that are given so freely. As I understand healing, it is impossible to be totally healed without some influence from each tool: the biomechanical, the mental, and the spiritual.

My Bias

Before I progress too far into this discussion I feel compelled to outline my bias. I am a Christian (big surprise there), and I believe in an omniscient and omnipotent God. I was raised Baptist, flunked out of Presbyterianism, and am now a recovering Methodist! Becoming a Methodist was more of an intuitive decision rather than one based on strict adherence to doctrine. I have found as I study more about John Wesley, the father of Methodism, that I share many of his beliefs regarding health and healing. Wesley wrote extensively about healing, the use of "natural" remedies, and the power of healing prayer. Many of my own beliefs are fostered by Wesley's treatises on the importance of healing the whole person, physically and spiritually. So I am initiating this discussion based on the firm belief that prayer is a wonderfully miraculous force for healing.

I am a physician, and as such I was trained to be analytical and logical in my approach to healing. I was taught that "first do no harm" meant: Don't subject a patient to any therapy that is either unproven or more hazardous than it is potentially beneficial. And I believe the majority of people want that kind of reassurance. People expect their health care provider to suggest treatments that are efficacious, practical, and safe. The old adage, "People don't care what you know as long as they know that you care," is true to a degree. I believe people do care that the person giving them advice about their health is competent, knowledgeable, and compassionate. Leaps of faith should be used sparingly in medicine, because if you leap indiscriminately you can land in some deep holes. It is with this background that I approached the study of prayer and healing.

Definitions

Healing, as I use the term, refers to much more than just ridding the body of disease. It goes back to the origin of the word haelan, which means to make whole. Whole in this sense is the balance between mind, body, and soul. I call this the healing triad, where each component is dependent on the other, and, to achieve balance, all parts must be in harmony. If one is out of balance, it can't help but influence another. In this concept, *health* is defined as achieving a balance in all three components. Simply getting rid of a sore throat with an antibiotic is only a small part of the health picture.

For true health one must look at diet, stress, relationships, and spiritual well-being, all of which may play a role in initiating, healing, or perpetuating that sore throat.

What does menopause mean to you? How do you view your own health status? These are important questions that you must answer to progress toward health in midlife and beyond. A study done at Harvard a few years back evaluated what factors were most predictive of death for a person in the next ten years. The results were surprising. It wasn't family history or past history. It wasn't even the presence of current health problems. The most predictive factor of a person's mortality in the ensuing ten years was their perception of their own health status. What was fascinating was that it didn't matter if they were right! In other words, these were people that by most criteria were considered unhealthy. However, if they themselves believed they were healthy individuals, they tended to be alive at the end of ten years. Those who felt they were in poor health even if they were healthy were also shown to influence their lifespan, but to a lesser degree. Our thoughts, feelings, and emotions can have a marked effect on our health, and are a crucial part of this balance.

I am not a theologian. That should be painfully obvious by now. My definition of prayer is simple. It is communication with God. Prayer can take many different forms. Many would assume that it is talking out loud in English to a patriarchal male with a long flowing beard, somewhere in the sky. That image and approach is OK, but this communication can be many other things. It can be songs or music, it can be dance, and it can be silence. It can be anything and anytime you and God are together, and that is all the time! This is the essence of what Paul meant when he entreated the Ephesians to "pray at all times and on every occasion in the power of the Holy Spirit. Stay alert and be persistent in your prayers for all Christians everywhere." (Ephesians 6:18)

Prayer can take place anytime and anywhere. When I run, I pray. As I run along the riverbank and the fog creeps down the river and the sun gushes over the treetops, I feel very close to God. The physical experience of running in God's beauty is overwhelming. I have had some real heart-to-heart talks with God on those long runs. Granted, at times I am praying, "God please let me make it back before I die of exhaustion!" But, for the most part, it is a joyful time alone with the Creator in which I establish a personal connection.

I was pleased to find that there are many others who share this idea of "prayerful activity." Linus Mundy founded a movement called Prayer Walking in 1985. He stated, "Action and contemplation have always been an American characteristic. By praying and walking at the same time, you really can get both spiritual and physical exercise."[1]

And remember, prayer is a dialogue. It is two-way communication. If you spend all of your time talking, how will you ever hear answers to your prayers? Think about building a relationship with your spouse. If you spent all your time talking and never listening to him, you wouldn't get to know him at all. So it is with God. How can you expect to build a relationship unless you hear Him talk? So you have to listen. Just being quiet is so important. Be still, be quiet, and be open.

As a physician who promotes healing on a daily basis, I am intrigued with the idea of incorporating prayer into my practice. Believing as I do, I *have* to incorporate prayer into my practice. I must pray for my patients. I wonder at times if I don't if it will be tantamount to malpractice. (I hope no attorneys are paying attention.) In order to successfully integrate these beliefs into a clinical practice, I began to ask questions.

Are prayer and science compatible? Can they coexist or are they mutually exclusive? Can prayer be tested? What is the evidence that prayer is an effective healing tool?

If I lived in the Inquisition, some church elders would be gathering the lighter fluid and marshmallows because they would burn me at the stake for asking such heretical questions. But these questions and many others must be answered before an integration of science and faith can be accomplished. Again let me reiterate that I know by faith that prayer heals. The issue is not about whether it does or doesn't.

The question arises, is the scientific method developed enough to validate this miraculous ability? Asking these questions doesn't weaken my faith; it strengthens it, and it affirms it. This is not about proving or disproving prayer, (I have trouble doing long division, and I'm not about to try to fully understand prayer). It is about showing the awesome power of the Creator in providing this glorious tool for us to employ. Dr. Larry Dossey, a Texas internist who has written extensively on the healing power of prayer, said, "When we test prayer we are not storming heaven's gates. These studies can be sacred reverent exercises. Testing prayer can actually be a form of worship, a ritual in which we express our gratitude for this remarkable phenomenon."[2]

The burden is on science to demonstrate the power of prayer. I know it works; can science confirm that? The person suffering from chronic pelvic pain is a patient that most gynecologists dread, mainly because the etiology of the pain is often so difficult to identify and even more troublesome to treat. The pain exists. The problem is being able to identify its source with available methods. Don't confuse the situation by thinking the reverse, "Well, if we can't identify the pain source, then the pain must be in her head." The same applies to prayer. We know prayer works by our faith. Can science demonstrate that?

If we are going to study prayer how are we going to define it? How do you measure prayer? What is a good outcome and what is not? Anyone attempting to look at the scientific evidence for prayer must address these critical issues. This is not bringing God into the laboratory; it is bringing the laboratory to God.

To answer these questions I did what physicians commonly do, I began a search of the medical literature. I was astounded by what I found. Not only have others asked these same questions, but they had also written profusely regarding it. The volume of literature on the healing power of prayer in legitimate scientific journals is astonishing.

One of the first studies I discovered was published by the *Southern Medical Journal* in 1989 by a cardiologist in San Francisco named

Dr. Randolph Byrd. He randomly assigned 393 patients admitted to the coronary care unit of his hospital to be in either a "prayed-for" group or a "non-prayed-for" group. These were very sick people as their admitting diagnosis was either a heart attack or a presumed heart attack. Neither the patients or the doctors or nurses knew who was in each group, so this was a randomized, double-blind study. The groups doing the praying were given the first names of the patients, their diagnosis, and their condition. The instructions the prayer groups were given were that they were asked to pray for a rapid recovery with few complications, and that the patients didn't die. It was interesting to note that the prayer groups were in San Francisco and other parts of the country.

The results were exciting. The "prayed-for" group was five times less likely to need antibiotics during their hospitalization and three times less likely to develop pulmonary edema. None of the "prayed-for" group required intubation (being placed on a ventilator) while twelve in the other group did. Fewer in the "prayed-for" group died, although this number was not statistically significant.[3] If this had been a new "wonder drug," the pharmaceutical companies would have been crawling all over themselves to patent it.

Because of the controversial nature of this study, it raised as many questions as it answered. Any good study does just that. This work laid the foundation for many other studies to follow.

The Byrd study was not without some legitimate criticism. Because Byrd was a Christian, many felt his use of only Christian prayer groups was part of a hidden agenda. Some believed it was an attempt to promote the idea that only "born-again" Christians had access to the holy hotline of healing. Others criticized what was called the first-name factor. Since the prayer groups were only given the first names of the patients, what would happen if there were two Johns, one in the "prayed-for" group and one in the "non-prayed-for" group? Outside prayer was not controlled for. In other words, there was no mechanism to track whether Aunt Sally organized a prayer group at her church for Uncle Joe, completely independent of the study. And what if Uncle Joe was in the "non-prayed-for" group?

In spite of the complaints and criticisms, many prominent physicians thought the study presented some valuable information. Dr. William Nolen, prominent surgeon and author, said, "It looks like this study will stand up to scrutiny . . . . Maybe we doctors ought to be writing on our order sheets, 'pray three times a day.' If it works. . . . It works."

Prayer In Nonhuman Systems

These criticisms illustrate the intrinsic difficulty in studying prayer in humans. There are so many factors, so many variables, so many individual variations that it is hard (if not impossible) to eliminate these variables and only look at the influence you are interested in: prayer, in this case.

The next logical step, given this difficulty, is to study prayer and its effects on nonhuman systems. The use of nonhuman subjects somewhat simplifies the design and increases the statistical validity. In many of those cases only the item you are interested in testing is changed. Again the literature on this approach is vast. It appears that there are even more published studies on prayer's healing ability on animals and plants than on people!

Dr. Dan Benor summarized the findings of many of these studies in a paper he authored. He reviewed 131 studies that specifically focused on prayer's effects on plants and animals, and in 56 he found statistically significant evidence of a positive impact on the organism.[4]

Anyone who is interested in this topic should get Larry Dossey's book *Healing Words*. He provides an excellent review of much of the scientific work dealing with prayer over the past decade.

After reviewing all the evidence I was haunted by two questions. If prayer works, why doesn't it always work? Why do spiritual people get sick? The answer to the first question lies in how I asked the question. What I was really asking was, if prayer works, why doesn't it always work *as I want it to*?

Are we so presumptuous to claim to know the mind of God? Can we begin to understand the purpose that God holds for all that exists in us? When prayer doesn't have the expected result, do we assume that God didn't hear or that we know better than the most perfect outcome? I suggest not. It is an expression of faith that we understand that all prayers are heard and answered. God answers prayers in ways that are not always congruent with our beliefs and demands. I am reminded of God's admonition to Job when questioned about His actions. "Are you going to discredit my justice and condemn me so you can say you are right? Are you as strong as God, and can you thunder with a voice like His?" (Job 40:8–9)

When we pray for someone to be healed, is it not better to pray for us to know how to help them be at peace with themselves and God? To me that is true healing. If we, as Christians, place death as an endpoint, if it represents a failure of healing prayer, then we are in for much disappointment. Death happens! It is a reality of the physical world we inhabit. As Christians, we don't view death as finality. Therefore it shouldn't be viewed as a failure of anything other than the cells that make up the body, not the soul.

Healing and Death

Think of the problems that would arise if everyone who was prayed for not to die, didn't. We would be living shoulder to shoulder, with little space to move. Death is a natural result of physical laws, yet it is not the gauge for the success or failure of prayer. One of my favorite sayings is "Eat healthy. Exercise daily. Die anyway!" That is a cynical way of viewing life, but it is steeped in truth. We all will die. I'm reminded of the man who died and went to heaven. Once there, it was more magnificent than he ever imagined. He said to St. Peter, "The songs, the beauty! If I had known it was going to be this great I would have come here years earlier."

St. Peter replied, "You would have if you hadn't eaten so many of those bran flakes!"

I am convinced that a person can die and be healed. Dan Richardson was a devoted Christian who lost his battle with cancer at an early age. This poem was read at his funeral. The author is unknown.

Cancer is so limited. . . .
It cannot cripple love,
It cannot shatter hope,
It cannot corrode faith,
It cannot eat away peace,
It cannot destroy confidence,
It cannot kill friendship,
It cannot shut out memories,
It cannot silence courage,
It cannot invade the soul
It cannot reduce eternal life,
It cannot quench the Spirit,
It cannot lessen the power of the resurrection.

You cannot tell me that this man was not healed! He may not have been in this world any longer, but his spirit soared.

The Healthy Christian

Why do spiritual people get sick? This is a question that many theologians have struggled with for centuries. The entire book of Job in the Bible addresses this question, among others. Disease and illness are, in large part, a matter of the natural consequences of our choices. If you smoke, your risk of lung cancer skyrockets. If you don't exercise and don't eat a healthy diet, you are more likely to succumb to heart disease. These are predictable outcomes to God's unyielding natural laws. There is not a one-to-one correlation between spirituality and health. There is no question that pursuing a spiritual, prayerful life will improve one's health (mind, body, and spirit) but it does not free you from disease. God is the great healer, but living a Christian life does not guarantee health.

Do I understand why young children get cancer? Can I make sense of the suffering of AIDS victims? Can I logically justfy why bad things happen to good people? No, I can't. But I can think about it, study about it, pray about it, and hope for comfort and understanding. Unlike the attempt of Steven Hawking, the physicist with Lou Gehrig's disease and author of *A Brief History of Time*, I do not profess to "know the mind of God." But I do know Paul's command in 1 Thessalonians 5:17: "Always be joyful. Keep on praying. *No matter what happens*, always be thankful, for this is God's will for you who belong to Christ Jesus" (emphasis mine).

There are numerous examples in a variety of faiths of spiritually aware persons who were physically afflicted. Buddha, arguably a very spiritual person, died of food poisoning. St. Bernadette, the girl who saw the visions of the Virgin Mary at Lourdes, died of bone cancer at age thirty-five. Suzuki Roshi, who introduced Zen Buddhism to the United States, succumbed to cancer of the liver.

The best example I have found of why bad things happen to good people is the story of Job. The book begins with the statement, "He was blameless, a man of complete integrity. He feared God and stayed away from evil." Yet tragedy after tragedy befell this spiritual man. What is the conclusion at the end of this story? It is easy to believe that we have all the answers. In reality, only God knows why things happen as they do, and we must always remember that He is in control. We are not puppets. We show our love and devotion by our decisions, however God's love is always there, guiding events. The Life Application Bible Commentary puts it this way:

> God is in control. In our world invaded by sin, calamity and suffering come to good and bad alike.
>
> This does not mean that God is indifferent, uncaring, unjust, or powerless to protect us. Bad things happen because we live in a fallen world, where both believers and unbelievers are hit with the tragic consequences of sin. God allows evil for a time although he turns it around for our good (Romans 8:28). We may have no answers as to why God allows evil, but we can be sure He is all-powerful and knows what he is doing. The next time you face trials and dilemmas, see them as opportunities to turn to God for strength. You will find a God who only desires to show His love and compassion to you. If you can trust Him in pain, confusion, and loneliness, you will win the victory and eliminate doubt, one of Satan's greatest footholds in your life. Make God your foundation. You can never be separated from His love.[5]

The Book of Job also illustrates that disease is not a punishment sent by God. It irritates me to hear people state that AIDS is God's revenge on the gay population. That is not only ignorant but dead wrong, and the Scriptures reinforce that. Look at John 9:1–3: "As Jesus was walking along, he saw a man who had been blind from birth. 'Teacher,' his disciples asked him, 'Why was this man born blind? Was it a result of his own sins or those of his parents?'

"It was not because of his sins or his parents' sins,' Jesus answered. 'He was born blind so the power of God could be seen in him."

The story continues as Jesus heals the blind man, fulfilling his destiny as an example of the healing power of Christ. If I imagine myself as the blind man and project his thoughts, I envision myself asking: Why me? Why was I born blind? Why do I have to suffer this affliction? Apparently the disciples were troubled by these same questions, and this prompted their quizzing the Messiah. It is obvious from the way the question is worded that they believed, as many did and still do, that the only understandable explanation for this man's infirmity lay in some defect in his or his parents' character. In other words, his blindness was a punishment for some unknown sin. Jesus quickly countered this belief by eloquently explaining that the blindness had nothing to do with sins or behavior. He stated that God knew the true meaning of this illness, and it was to illuminate the glory of God through the healing.

Dr. Larry Dossey states, "Sickly saints and healthy sinners show us that there is no invariable, one-to-one relationship between one's level of spiritual attainment and the degree of one's physical health. It is obvious that one can achieve great spiritual heights and still get very sick."[6] Remember, healing is much more than just ridding the body of disease; it is balancing mind, body, and spirit.

Fruits of Prayer

What benefits do we see in prayer? If we don't know or can't predict results, then why pray? In simple terms, it's not about getting. It is about learning to achieve a state of prayerfulness—a state where you become open to God's love and healing presence. Jane

Vennard, in an audio tape called "Intercessory Prayer," talks about the "fruits" of prayer.[7] I love the analogy of fruit because it is a substance that must be cultivated and nourished to grow, and in turn can serve. as nourishment to others. Fully developed, it can even seed the growth of additional fruit. She states that one of these fruits of prayer is a God-centered existence. God is responsible for all we are, have, and will be, and through prayer we remind ourselves of that. Praying for healing will refocus us on the Healer instead of the disease. It puts God in the center of our lives and encourages us to replace our egocentric thoughts with those of divine grace.

The second fruit of healing prayer is compassion. Through prayer we embrace a heightened level of compassion for those about whom we pray. This takes the form of empathy, truly feeling the needs of the afflicted. Healing prayer brings hope. When people who survived suicide attempts are interviewed, inevitably they report reaching a state of hopelessness. There is no greater feeling of desperation than being without hope. Praying for yourself or others restores hope, perpetuates hope, and in some cases creates hope.

Ms. Vennard states that another fruit of intercessory prayer is action. Whether it is serving meals to the homeless or helping a tornado victim find parts of their ravaged home, prayer can spur us to action. The action itself may be a form of prayer. We may join a protest for basic human rights or volunteer at a hospice. Prayer gives us direction; it provides focus. Listen, listen, and listen. In the silence of prayer, the call to action can be deafening.

Finally, prayer emphasizes thankfulness, the attitude of gratitude. Giving thanks to God for healing reminds us where the healing originates. It is a simple concept, but one I find helpful in centering my faith. It is a statement of faith. I believe; therefore, I thank and praise. Only a fool would thank someone for something they knew they wouldn't receive.

How To

Richard Foster, in his book *Prayer*, says, "God, I have a thousand arguments against healing prayer. You are the one argument for it. . . .

you win!"[8] He then explains his approach to praying for healing. He says this is not a "how to" guide for healing prayer, but a template to build on. I have found his ideas useful as a guide to help in all communications with God, not just specific to healing. He describes four steps to healing prayer: listening, asking, knowing, and thanking.

Listening is vital to effective communication, with God or anyone else. God gave us two ears and one mouth in the hopes that we would listen twice as much as we talked! How strange that in prayer so often we focus on one side of the dialogue. One of the monumental apprehensions people have about prayer is "doing it right." They are afraid that they will not say the right thing or even know what to say. You cannot pray wrong! Just the act of praying makes it right. You don't have to say anything! Just be quiet and listen. This may be more difficult for some than speaking.

Being quiet does not come naturally for many people. But listening can be a learned behavior. Listen to people, and they will tell you their prayer needs. First year medical students are told that simply listening to patients will provide the diagnosis of their problem the vast majority of times. Practice being still in prayer. It will take the pressure off, and you may be surprised at what you hear. In his book, Richard Foster talks about his own intercessory prayer experience. He says, "After prayer for my immediate family, I wait quietly until individuals or situations spontaneously rise to my awareness. I then offer these to God, listening to see if any special discernment comes to guide the content of the prayer."[9]

Ask God for healing for yourself and others. God knows your needs, so this is not attempting to relay new information. Rather, asking is both an act of faith and a reminder of the needs of others. By asking, you crystallize your thoughts and focus on what is important. When we become clear on the needs, asking invites healing to emerge. It opens our hearts and minds to the healing love that is always right there. It is OK to ask.

Msgr. Arthur Tonne relates the story of a mother who told her young son to go to bed and be sure to say his prayers and ask God to make him a good boy. The boy's father, passing by the bedroom, overheard his son praying: "And God make me a good boy if You can; and if You can't, don't worry about it, 'cause I'm having fun the way I am."

God wants us to ask. Jesus said, "Keep on asking, and you will be given what you ask for. Keep on looking, and you will find. Keep on knocking, and the door will be opened. For everyone who asks, receives. Everyone who seeks, finds. And the door is opened to everyone who knocks." (Matt 7:7–8)

A well-known motivational speaker's favorite phrase is "Know your outcome." Here "know" is much more than a belief. It is that feeling that starts in the bottom of your toes and slowly fills every molecule of your being. We know with our whole person: body, mind, and spirit. This is a step of assurance. In this sense it is almost analogous to faith. "What is faith? It is the confident assurance [knowing] that what we hope for is going to happen. It is the evidence of things we cannot yet see" (Heb. 11:1). And Peter writes, "Knowing God leads to self-control. Self-control leads to patient endurance, and patient endurance leads to godliness" (2 Pet. 1:6).

The final step is thanks, the attitude of gratitude. Giving thanks for what we know is to be. Praise and prayer are like peanut butter and jelly; they just go together! David knew how to give thanks:

Praise the Lord!

How good it is to sing praises to our God!
How delightful and how right!
    The LORD is rebuilding Jerusalem
and bringing the exiles back to Israel.
He heals the brokenhearted,
binding up their wounds.
    He counts the stars and
calls them all by name.
How great is our Lord! His power is absolute!
His understanding is beyond comprehension!
The LORD supports the humble,
but He brings the wicked down into the dust.
Sing out your thanks to the LORD;
sing praises to our God, accompanied by harps. (Ps. 147:1–7)

Prayer Works

Emily and Stan, a young couple, were expecting their second child. Their firstborn was five-year-old Sammy. Sammy would crawl up next to his mother and rub her ever-expanding tummy and sing to his future sibling. It was his way of getting to know the unborn baby. This continued throughout the uneventful pregnancy until labor ensued. The labor was short, yet at the end Emily developed some problems that necessitated an emergency C-section.

The joy and anticipation of the new arrival was somewhat dampened by the news that the new baby girl showed signs of an infection. The little girl, whom they named Sally, was taken to the neonatal intensive care nursery in this small hospital to be watched closer. After a few hours the pediatrician came to Emily's room and told her that the little baby had taken a turn for the worse. They were going to have to transfer the baby to a specialized nursery downtown for more intensive care. You can only imagine the devastation and apprehension both Emily and Stan felt as they watched their newborn being wheeled into the ambulance for the transfer.

After a day at the new hospital, the neonatologist spoke to Emily as she was visiting Sally. "We are very concerned about Sally," he said slowly. "The next twenty-four hours are critical, she could turn around or she could get a lot worse. I just thought you should know to be able to tell any family members to stay close by."

Emily could read between the lines. She knew that the doctor was telling her that her child might not make it. Then it occurred to her that Sammy had not yet seen his baby sister. She decided that if there was a chance that baby Sally was not going to make it, she had to get Sammy in to see her.

The neonatal intensive care unit is a very mechanical, sterile environment and small children are not allowed to visit because of the risk of infection. This didn't dissuade Emily as she dressed Sammy in a little rolled up scrub suit and put on a mask and walked into the unit. The nurses went berserk! But when they realized what was going on they reluctantly agreed to the brief visit. Babies in a NICU lie in beds that are up on pedestals to allow the nurses to work with them more easily. They retrieved a couple of boxes for Sammy to stand on, and he climbed up and peered over the bassinet for a first look at his new sister.

To most, the sight of a little baby with a tube in her throat and IV lines from her arms would be frightening. Not to Sammy. He peered intently at Sally and then spontaneously reached down and grabbed her tiny hand . . . and began to sing, just as he had done to his mommy's tummy. "You are my sunshine, my only sunshine. You make me happy when skies are gray. You'll never know, dear, how much I love you. Please, God, don't take my sister away."

The nurses were the first to notice a difference in the baby. That evening Sally's vital signs stabilized and her temperature became normal. She was able to breath on her own within twenty-four hours and was discharged home two days later, a healthy happy baby sister. The local newspaper that had followed the story called it a miracle; the doctors and nurses all called it a miracle. I call it the healing power of prayer.

CHAPTER FOURTEEN

Frequently Asked Questions

Am I going crazy?

If I kept a tally of commonly asked questions, this would rank at or near the top. Not a day goes by that somebody doesn't pose this rhetorical question. It is often a springboard for women to introduce a discussion of PMS or menopause. Let me reassure you that you are not a candidate for the straightjacket. That is not to say that at times you do not feel like you are losing it, because you do. Many women who suffer from PMS or perimenopausal symptoms struggle with a sense of loss of control. "This is not like me. . . . I don't normally do these kind of things." This perceived loss of control creates the illusion of being less than sane. Granted, there are physiological changes that are manifested in "crazy" feelings, yet for the vast majority of women, these feelings are normal and transient. You are not going crazy; you are going through change. And with change come different emotions, reactions, and perceptions, all of which are normal adaptive behaviors.

Is it normal to have irregular periods?

This is often the first sign of hormonal changes. The menstrual cycle is a delicate balance of many parts in which any change in any player can disrupt the entire cycle. The most common scenario is where the cycle lengths initially shorten and then actually start to spread out. It is not unusual for a woman to have periods every two to three weeks for a time and then see the menses begin to skip months. The amount of the flow can vary tremendously. It can be anywhere from a little spotting to a flood. It is hard to give any accurate predictions for a specific woman, as the actual experience is so individualized. Suffice it to say that, in the perimenopause, the cycle can masquerade as almost anything.

Why am I gaining weight?

One of the most prevalent myths of menopause is that every woman gains weight because of the hormone changes. The battle cry of the menopausal woman is "I don't want to get fat and hairy!" The reality is that both these fears are unfounded. Demographic studies show that the average woman puts on more weight in her thirties than in her fifties. This myth is largely perpetuated by the known association of weight gain with HRT. However, just being menopausal doesn't make you fat. Caloric requirements decrease with age, so you must compensate appropriately. Staying active and eating well can maintain weight in the menopause as well as in any other generation. If you are gaining weight in the menopause, check your activity level and your dinner plate.

Do all women need hormones?

No. Just as I wouldn't give all women insulin to prevent the possible deterioration brought about by high blood sugar, so I wouldn't give all women hormone replacement to thwart the ravages of aging. First of all, it won't do that and second, hormones are not innocuous substances. There are very specific indications for HRT, and only when the benefits outweigh the risks should HRT be considered. Many women do benefit from HRT; however, there are alternatives. Being female and over fifty does not automatically place you on the hormone fast track.

How do I know if I am in menopause?

The most common indication is the lack of menses. If you go six months and don't have a period (and are not pregnant and have no other hormone irregularity) then you are in menopause. A few simple blood tests (FSH, LH) may help further define your hormonal status. Don't forget about the importance of symptoms in the perimenopause. In fact, this time is often defined by the appearance of symptoms.

Why did my sex drive drive off?

Libido is a complex drive. Many factors contribute to sexual appetite. Another myth surrounding menopause is that sex is about as much fun as a screen door on a submarine. This is a damaging belief, and, for many, just the opposite is true. A recent survey showed over 50 percent of menopausal women actually feel their sexual functioning is better now than it was when they were younger. So blaming menopause for declining sex drive is often misguided and obstructs other causes. There is a hormonal component to libido, and conditions such as atrophic vaginitis can inhibit functionality and enjoyment, yet many can and do enjoy mutually satisfying sexuality in the golden years. If you are not one of these fortunate women, look at all aspects before blaming hormones.

Do hormones cause cancer?

When women ask this, they are most commonly referring to estrogen and breast cancer. However, the only cancer that has been definitively linked to estrogen use is cancer of the uterus (endometrial). Using estrogen alone over an extended period of time unquestionably increases your risk of uterine cancer when compared to the general population. Using a progestigen with the estrogen in a proper dose essentially eliminates this increased risk. The vast majority of studies do not show a direct cause and effect between estrogen use and breast cancer. There is epidemiological data that suggests that estrogen may act as a promoter of breast cancer in susceptible women. In other words, it acts like a fertilizer. It doesn't initiate a cancer, but if one develops, it can accelerate its growth. There have been no links of estrogen with other female cancers such as ovarian or cervical.

If I take hormones, do I stay on them forever?

It depends entirely on the rationale for taking them in the first place. Step number one is being absolutely sure why you are using hormones. There are basically two reasons, symptom relief or long-term prophylactic benefits (for example, osteoporosis prevention and reduction of heart disease). Symptoms such as hot flashes and skin changes are often transient. On average these physiological changes may persist for two to three years. Many women take HRT during this time to abate these problems and then stop the hormones. Their symptoms never return. If this were the only reason for the HRT use, then it would no longer be necessary. On the other hand, if the primary motive for using HRT is the long-term health benefits, then a longer course of treatment is warranted. Studies indicate that the long-term benefits evaporate after about six months of being off the HRT. Assess your individual needs and discuss this with your doctor.

If I have had a hysterectomy, do I still need a Pap smear?

A Pap smear is designed to detect precancerous cells from the cervix. The vast majority of women who have had a hysterectomy had their cervix removed also (it is the part of the uterus that projects into the vagina). Do in that respect they have no risk of cervical cancer. However, the Pap can give information about the remaining vaginal cells. I have seen the rare woman who has precancerous cells of the vagina that were detected by the Pap smear. Also the Pap can help assess the hormonal status of the vaginal tissue and can occasionally detect an infection. The insurance companies will tell you that a yearly Pap for a woman who has had a hysterectomy is not cost-effective, yet I believe they are wrong. Much more than just a

Pap is accomplished at a yearly visit. This is a time for an overall health maintenance checkup. There are many issues such as breast exams, evaluation of the ovaries, and stress management that should be addressed at this yearly visit. Without the ritual of the Pap smear many women would not seek regular checkups, and many opportunities for prevention would be missed.

When should I get a mammogram?

The debate rages about the proper time to begin mammography and the ideal interval between mammograms. This will never be resolved, because there is no definite answer. All we can do is make recommendations based on large population studies that give us the highest likelihood of detecting an early cancer. Mammography, like most technology, is imperfect and will miss cancers. Our job is to try to minimize those and limit the number of false positive findings. There are no cookbook answers, and each woman must examine her risk factors and consult with her health care worker to determine an appropriate screening schedule that meets her needs. I am much more aggressive about getting early and frequent mammograms in women with a strong family history (mother or sister with breast cancer, especially before the age of fifty). Getting a baseline mammogram between ages thirty-five and forty is reasonable, and following this with one every two years until age fifty is a safe routine. Yearly mammograms after the age of fifty are a must! I have seen many early cancers that were detected by routine mammography long before the woman or I could feel any changes.

How much calcium should I take?

Calcium is an essential mineral in bone metabolism. The postmenopausal women should consume 1,200-1,500 mg calcium a day to optimize her bone health. With the average standard American diet most women will consume between 700-1,000 mg a day. Most women after fifty should either increase their calcium intake in their diet or supplement with 500-800 mg a day. This is especially important for those at high risk for osteoporosis, or who have certain dietary restrictions (for example, lactose intolerance). You may have to experiment with the type of calcium to find a form that doesn't bother your gastrointestinal tract.

What is the best exercise for PMS and menopause?

There is no "best." The important point is just doing something. The best type of exercise for you is dependent on what you want to accomplish. In general, aerobic forms of exercise are the best for overall fitness and weight loss. Walking at a brisk pace for thirty to forty-five minutes at least three times a week is generally accepted as the simplest and most effective approach for the novice exerciser. This is not to say that walking is only for beginners! My wife is a long-time exerciser, and she uses walking as her cornerstone activity. Done at the right pace and for the right amount of time, walking can be a fabulous workout.

If I am on hormones will I continue to have periods?

Most women using both estrogen and progestigens, who still have a uterus, will continue to have periods. These are artificially created by the interaction of the hormones on the uterine lining. If you are truly menopausal, then resuming periods with HRT will not make you more likely to be fertile. Alternative ways of dosing HRT can elicit different bleeding patterns, and many have gone to a continuous regimen that eliminates periods in about 60 percent of women.

Is herb use New Age or anti-Christian?

Part of my motivation for writing this book was to explode the myth that the use of herbs and alternative approaches to certain problems was exclusive to New Age practitioners. The use of oils, herbs, and balms is richly embedded in both Old and New Testament writings. The confusion arises in the association of herbal use with some Eastern philosophies. Herbs and foodstuffs were used as medicines in many Eastern societies for thousands of years. They became intertwined in the cultural milieu of the times, and this association has persisted. Granted, many alternative practitioners incorporate mysticism, New Age philosophy, and non-Christian beliefs in their therapies—but don't confuse the messenger with the message. A Christian woman should embrace herbs, foods, and vitamins as God-given tools for health and well-being.

I used an herbal remedy for hot flashes and it did nothing, why?

Just as not all prescription medicines will work for all people, so herbs will not be effective for some. I have found that many of the "failures" with herbal and nutritional therapies are actually due to improper dosing or duration of use. These treatments do not work overnight. Many may take two to three months to exert their effect. However, there will be those who do not respond to a particular therapy. Luckily there are usually reasonable alternatives. Don't be disillusioned if your first option doesn't accomplish what you desire. Try others.

Why doesn't my doctor talk about herbs or alternative treatment programs?

For many it is simply unfamiliar territory, and they are actually doing you a favor by not offering something they know little about. Hopefully, they will be encouraging and supportive of your efforts and open to working with you. This stuff is not taught in medical school. Unless doctors have an interest themselves and have done a great deal of independent study, they probably will either say they know nothing about nutraceuticals or downplay their effectiveness. Some medical schools are incorporating coursework in alternative and complementary approaches to their curriculum. This will serve to expand the numbers of physicians who have a foundational knowledge of these practices. Naturopaths, homeopaths, herbalists, and alternative practitioners by nature focus more on these subjects as a part of their training. In turn, these professionals can lack the balance and knowledge of more mainstream methods of healing.

How long does menopause last?

Menopause means only one thing, and that is the cessation of the menses. So in that respect, it is impossible to put a time frame on its duration. When women ask this, they are usually asking how long symptoms will continue. This varies from none at all to several years.

On average, a woman can expect to experience hot flashes for two to three years after her period stops. The other symptoms are so varied that there is no "average" length.

Live the Mission

Who, am. I really? Where do I want to be in five years? What is my mission? What is my purpose and vision? Do I want to live as I am now, or do I want something different? Does God have a mission for my life?

Proverbs says that "a people without vision will surely perish". A vision is knowledge of what you want to be, accomplish, and understand. To know your outcome is to see the path to your vision. Imagine how difficult it would be to plan a weeklong trip or vacation and not know your destination. You wouldn't know how long to allot for travel. You wouldn't know where to make nighttime hotel reservations. You wouldn't even know which way to turn out of the driveway.

So it is with life. If you don't have a clear picture of where you want to go, you will be relegated to wandering, aimlessly searching for an unclear, unidentified destination. If you do not have an acute understanding of what you want your life to be, then you can imagine the absurdity and frustration of living day-to-day without purpose.

Do you know how you want to spend this third of your life called menopause? Have you envisioned how this time, whether you are in your forties dealing with PMS or later in perimenopause, can be a celebration rather than a struggle to survive?

I challenge you to begin today to create the vision of a fulfilling and purposeful life. This first step is essential, for it creates the atmosphere in which all your thoughts, actions, and beliefs will be nurtured. Saturate this vision with prayer. Let prayer be the canvas on which you paint your midlife. No matter the form, color, or style of the picture, the canvas is always there, underlying every stroke, supporting every dream.

Mission and purpose can come in prayer. It can come through action, reading, meditation, and discussion. How one formulates his or her mission is unique, yet I find the common denominator is prayer. Missions are not complicated. Jesus said, "I came that they may have life and have it abundantly." Nehemiah's goal was simply to rebuild the wall of Jerusalem. The twelve apostles shared a common mission to go out and teach what they had learned. Mother Teresa's purpose was to show love and compassion to the poor. Your mission can be just as simple and no less grand.

This book is a springboard. It is meant to be a place to start. Neither I, nor anyone else, can determine how or if you use any of the information contained in these pages. My heartfelt prayer is that you will find some morsel of truth, some kernel of wisdom, to stimulate you to think and act. But don't stop there. This is just a beginning. This is only a door that opens to a vast storehouse of discoveries awaiting you on your journey.

Dr. Wayne Sotile, speaker and author, talks about stress in his book *Supercouple Syndrome*. He feels many of us live in times of high stress and low control. This is a toxic stress that can overwhelm our physical and spiritual well-being. This certainly describes the menopause for many women, a time of many stresses and loss of control. In fact, this scenario is associated with the highest rate of divorce, illness, and depression for women.

Take a close look at the idea of high stress/low control with respect to PMS and menopause. What I find interesting (and what I hope you understand after reading this book) is that both of these situations–high stress and low control–are situations that are influenced by your thoughts. You have already seen how stress is based on your perceptions. What is stressful to one may not be stressful to another; the difference is how each person perceives the stressor. The loss of control during PMS and menopause is often secondary to ignorance of choices and a lack of understanding of physiology. I have shown you how to take back control in the preceding chapters. You have guidelines to reshape your perception of stress and control, and you can alter the reality of your situation. But it starts with knowing where you are going. That often is determined by answering the "why" questions at the beginning of this chapter. If you can determine the "why," then the "how" will follow.

We've discussed one path to a celebration of midlife: Attitude, Aptitude, Action, and Apothecary. Begin with the intention of knowing your outcome. Know that God has a plan, and He will see you through. Be open to His guidance. Immerse yourself in prayer and meditation to determine your path. Listen. Hear God. Cultivate a personal friendship with Him. Educate yourself. Use every resource available to know options and to make decisions. Bathe yourself in knowledge and wisdom from the Word, friends, family, doctors, books, seminars, tapes, and experience. Make it an adventure! Take action. Use the knowledge that you acquire. Faith without works is dead, and, likewise, knowledge without action is impotent. Embrace exercise, vitamins, herbs, and healthy diets, and eliminate those behaviors you know to be harmful.

Enjoy life and all that is here for you. That implies action and commitment. This book is a call to action. It is a challenge to do something that, furthers your relationship with God and yourself. Immobility, inaction, stagnation, paralysis, and numbness are your enemies.

Every action begins with a thought. Every great deed and every whisper is predicated on a conviction. The only true failure in life is the person who takes no action, tries nothing new, or fears success. When you do something to better your feelings, thoughts, or emotions there are only two possible outcomes. Either you accomplish your task or you don't. And if you don't, you haven't failed. You have just learned another way not to get the results you want!

Everyone is unique. There are no two women who will waltz through midlife with the same dance steps. Each dance is special and your own. It stands to reason that not all women will benefit from every technique or recommendation in this book. This variation does not invalidate the suggestions. Take what feels right to you, try it, and evaluate whether it is accomplishing your goal. Is it eliminating the hot flashes? If not, try something else. Don't relinquish all other options. God will not abandon you, no matter what road you take.

To create a space for joy in the menopause or PMS, do the following:

1. *Make a plan; set a goal.* Decide where you want your life to go. Suffuse the process with prayer. There is nothing fiendish in visualizing the kind of life you want. Trust in God to open your heart and mind to the possibilities. He came in the person of Jesus so that you may have life and have it *abundantly*. Listen, believe, meditate, visualize, and pray.
2. *Don't lose sight of your mission.* It is so easy to get caught up in the hurry sickness of our times. Pay the bills. Drive the carpool. Climb the ladder. Volunteer here. Hurry over there. Every decision of importance you make should be measured by the standard of your vision. Doesthis action bring me closer to God? Does this activity support my calling?
3. *Remember that taking action drives the engine of happiness*. I suppose some could be content spending hours doing nothing. As I said earlier, a little loafing every now and then is refreshing, but it is not an effective lifestyle. The evidence is overwhelming that if you want to live a long and happy life you must stay active, both mentally and physically. The realities of aging place some limits, yet the greatest limiting factor is that which we place on ourselves.
4. *Constantly evaluate what you are doing*. Is this herb working? Is my prayer life what I want it to be? Am I losing the weight I want to? Do I sleep better at night? Never stop asking questions. Always reassess every major decision to see if it (a)

accomplishes the intended goal and (b) is consistent with your beliefs and integrity. If it is not getting you where you want to be, change course. Do something different; try a new angle. There are no failures, just different ways of doing things.

5. *Listen to others with a discerning ear.* A fool hears only what she wants to and nothing she should. When the student is ready the teacher will appear. Understand that most information you receive from the media has an agenda. It may be a positive spiritually-driven agenda, but a bias always exists. Be open, but be critical.
6. *Partner with someone; be it your spouse, a good friend, a support group, or your doctor.* Share your mission and your vision for this transition time and beyond. They will keep you accountable and will be supportive during the inevitable trials and tribulations.
7. *Have fun!* Don't ever underestimate the healing potential of good times. Laughter truly can be wonderful medicine. Norman Cousins knew it, Patch Adams knew it, and Slomon knew it. Now you know it, so laugh three times a day. Doctor's orders!
8. *Respect the healing triad: mind, body, and spirit.* Health means wholeness, and wholeness is a balance of all three. Remember the mobile, where none is isolated and each one exerts its influence on the other.
9. *Never stop learning.* I am continually amazed (but not surprised) at how much I don't know! It used to bother me, but now I see it as a glorious opportunity to discover. Never stop saying, "Ah-ha." Recapture the wonder of childhood where every day is an adventure.
10. *Always maintain the attitude of gratitude.* Thank God at every opportunity for blessing you with life and the ability to make it a wondrous journey. All we are and can be comes from God, and He even gave us an example to follow. Even in the darkest hours, even in the lowest points, even in the hottest flashes, He is there saying, "Come on, Sally. Come on, Julie. Come on, Barbara. Walk with me."

ENDNOTES

Introduction

1. B. Ettinger, D. K. Li, and R. Klien, "Continuation of postmenopausal hormone replacement therapy in cyclic and continuous regimens," *Menopause* 3 (1996): 185–89.
2. S. I. McMillen, *None of These Diseases* (GrandRapids, Mich.: Baker Book House, 1963), 15.
3. Ibid., 15.

Chapter One

1. G. Sheehy, *The Silent Passage*, rev. ed. (New York: Random House, 1998) author notes, 1.
2. J. Archer, "Relationship between Estrogen, Serotonin, and Depression," *Menopause* 6 (1999): 77.
3. F. Kostreski, article published in OB–Gyn News, December 15, 1998, 6.

Chapter Two

1. Owen, *Daughters of Eve* (Colorado Springs, Colorado: NavPress, 1995), 8.
2. E. B. Holifield, *Health and Medicine in the Methodist Tradition* (New York: Crossroad Publishers, 1986), p. 6.
3. M. Albom, *Tuesdays with Morrie* (New York: Doubleday, 1997), 43.
4. Ibid., 57.

Chapter Four

1. G. E. Abraham, "Nutritional factors in the etiology of premenstrual tension syndrome," *J of Reprod Med* 28 (1983): 446–64.
2. R. V. Norris and C. Sullivan, *PMS-premenstrual syndrome* (New York: Berkley Publishing, 1983).
3. M. Murray and J. Pizzorno, *Encyclopedia of Natural Medicine* (Rocklin, Calif.: Prima Health, 1998).
4. R. Russell, *What the Bible Says about Healthy Living* (Ventura, Calif.: Regal Books, 1996), 27.
5. D. Y. Jones, "Influence of dietary fat on self reporting menstrual symptoms," *Physiol Behav* 40 (1987): 483–7.
6. C. Longcope et al., "The effect of a low fat diet on estrogen metabolism," *J of CLin EndocrinoL Metab* 64 (1987): 1246–50.
7. Norris and Sullivan, PMS-premenstrual syndrome, 206.
8. U. Erasmus, *Fats that Heal, Fats that Kill* (B. C. Burnaby: Alive Books, 1994), 4.
9. Russell, *What the Bible Says about Healthy Living*, 178.
10. W Borr, "Pyridoxine supplements in the premenstrual syndrome," *Practitioner* 228 (1984): 425–27.
11. J. Klijnen, G. Teriet and P Ktiipschild, "Vitamin B6 in the treatment of PMS: a review," *Br J Obstet Gynaecol* 97 (1990): 847–52.
12. R. S. London et al., "The effect of alphatocopherol on premenstrual symptomatology: a double blind study," *J Amer Col Nutr* 3 (1984): 351-56.
13. S. Thys-Jacobs et al., "Calcium supplementation in premenstrual syndrome: a randomized cross over trial," *J Ger Intern Med* 4 (1989): 183-89.
14. J. G. Penland and P E. Johnson, "Dietary calcium and manganese effects on menstrual cycle symptoms," *Am J Obstet Gynecol* 168 (1993): 1417-23.

15. S. Thys-Jacobs et al., "Calcium carbonate and the premenstrual syndrome," *Am J Obstet Gynecol* (1998): 179.
16. C. Posacki, et al., "Plasma copper, zinc, and magnesium levels in patients with premenstrual tension syndrome," *Acta Obstet Gynecol Scand* 73 (1994): 452–55.
17. F. Facchinetti, "Oral magnesium successfully relieves premenstrual mood changes," *Obstet Gynecol* 78 (1991): 177–81.
18. A. Stewart, "Clinical and biochemical effects of nutritional supplementation of the premenstrual syndrome," *J Reprod Med* 32 (1987): 435–41.
19. P Y. Choi and P Salmon, "Symptom changes across the menstrual cycle in competitive sports, exercisers and sedentary women," *Br J Clin Psychol* 34 (1995): 447–60.
20. C. Bailey, *Smart Exercise* (New York: Houghton Mifflin, 1994), 273.
21. Ibid., 272.
22. B. Delaney and S. Delaney, quote from *Christian Reader* 33 no. 2.
23. J. Kabat-Zinn, *Full Catastrophe Living* (New York: Dell Publishing, 1990), 241.
24. H. C. H. Vogel, *The Nature Doctor* (New Canaan, Conn.: Keats Publishing, 1991).
25. *PDR for Herbal Medicines* (Montvale, N.J.: Medical Economics. 1998).
26. R. V. Farese et al., "Licorrice induced hypermineralcorticoidism," *N Eng J Med* 325 (1991): 1223–7.
27. C. Peleres-Welte and M. Albrecht, "Menstrual abnormalities and PMS: Vitus Agnus," *Therapiewoche Gynakol* 7 (1994): 49–52.

Chapter Five

1. N. Wright, *Simplify Your Life* (Wheaton, Ill.: Tyndale House, 1997), 6.
2. L. B. Jones, *Jesus CEO* (New York: Hyperion, 1995), 23.
3. N. Warren, *Finding Contentment* (Nashville: Thomas Nelson Publishers, 1997).

Chapter Six

1. Brilliant, quote from speech in 1978.
2. M. Lucado, *He Still Moves Stones* (Dallas: Word Publishing, 1993).

Chapter Seven

1. C. Swindoll, quoted from *Christian Reader* 33 no. 4.
2. B. Phillips, *Phillips Book of Great Thoughts and Funny Sayings* (Wheaton, Ill.: Tyndale House, 1993), 28.
3. Men of Integrity newsletter, 2 no. 2 (1997).
4. B. Johnson, *Living Somewhere Between Estrogen and Death* (Dallas: Word Publishing, 1997).

Chapter Eight

1. Collaborative Group on Hormonal Factors in Breast Cancer, *The Lancet* 350 (1997): 1047.
2. B. C. Arstomy, "Oestrogen Therapy after menopause," *Medj Aust* 148, no. 5 (1988): 213–14.
3. W. D. Dupont et al., "Menopausal estrogen replacement therapy and breast cancer," *Arch Intern Med* 151 (1991): 67–72.
4. K. K. Steinberg, "A meta analysis of the effect of estrogen replacement therapy on the risk of breast cancer," *JAMA* 265 (1991): 1985–90.
5. G. A. Colditz, "Hormone replacement therapy and the risk of breast cancer: results from epidemiological studies," *Am J Obstet Gynecol* 168 (1993): 1473–80.
6. J. L. Stanford et al., "Combined estrogen and progesterone replacement therapy in relation to risk of breast cancer in middle age women," *JAMA* 274 (1989): 137-42: D. W Kaufman, "Estrogen replacement therapy and the risk of breast cancer: results from the case controlled surveillance study," *Am J Epidemiol* 134 (1991): 1375–85: and J. R. Palmer et al., "Breast cancer risk after estrogen replacement therapy: results from the Toronto breast cancer study," *Am J Epidemiol* 134 (1991): 1386–95.
7. Colditz, "Hormone replacement therapy," 1473–80.
8. The writing group of the PEPI trial, "Effect of estrogen on heart disease risk factors in postmenopausal women: The postmenopausal estrogen/progesterone interventions trial," *JAMA* 273 (1995): 199–208.
9. Ibid.

Chapter Nine

1. Lotke and Albertazzi, "The effect of dietary soy supplementation on hot flushes," *Obstet Gynecoll* (1998): 6–11.
2. Ibid.
3. Messina, "The role of soy products in reducing cancer," *J National Cancer Institute* 83 (1991): 541–46.
4. J. W. Anderson, "Meta analysis on the effects of Soy protein intake on serum lipids," *N Eng J Med* 353 (1995): 276–82.
5. Aldercreutz, "Phytoestrogens in western diseases," Annuls of Medicine 29 (1997): 95–120.
6. R. S. Finkler, "The effect of vitamin E in the menopause," *J Clin Endocrinol Metab* 9 (1949): 89–94.
7. S. Lieberman, "A review of the effectiveness of Cimicifuga Racemosa for the symptoms of menopause," *J Women's Health* 5 (1998): 529.
8. W. Stoll, "Phytopharmacuetical influences on atrophic vaginal epithelium," Therapeuticum 1 (1987): 23–31: Wameche, "Influencing menopausal symptoms with a phytotherapeutic agent," *Med Welt* 36 (1985): 871–74.
9. E. Lehmann-Willenbrock and H. H. Riedel, "Clinical and endocrinological examinations concerning therapy of climacteric symptoms following hysterectomy with remaining ovaries," *Zentralbl Gynakol* 110 (1998): 611–18.
10. Warneche, "Influencing menopausal symptoms."
11. N. Beuscher, "Cimicifuga Racemosa," *Phytotherapie* 16 (1995): 301–10.
12. Stoll, "Phytopharmacuetical influences."
13. C. H. Folkins and W E. Sime, "Physical fitness training and mental health," *Am Psychologist* 36 (1981): 375–88.
14. C. Bailey, *Smart Exercise*, (New York: Houghton Mifflin, 1994), 271.
15. W. Poldinger, Calanchini, and W Scwartz, "A functional dimensional approach to depression: serotonin deficiency as a target syndrome in a comparison of 5-HTP and fluvoxamine," *Psychopathology* 24 (1991): 53–81.
16. Murray, Encyclopedia of Natural Medicine, 397.
17. E. V. Vorbach, W D. Hubner, and K. H. Arnoldt, "Effectiveness and tolerance of the Hypericumextract LI 160 in comparison with Imipramine: randomized double-blind study with 135 outpatients," *J Geriatr Psychiatry Neurol* 17 (1994): 519–23.

18. I. Hindmarch and Z. Subhan, "The psychopharmalogical effects of Ginkgo Biloba extract in normal healthy volunteers," *Int J Clin Pharmacol Res* 4 (1984): 89–93.

19. K. Linde, G. Ramirez, and C. D. Mulrow, "St. John's Wort for depression: an overview and meta analysis of randomized clinical trials," *Br Med J* 313 (1996): 253–58.

20. P. L. Lebars et al., "A placebo controlled double blind randomized trial of an extract of Gingko Biloba for dementia," *JAMA* 278 (1997): 1327–32.

21. M. S. Santos, F Ferreira, and A. P Cunha, "An liquid extract of valerian influences the transport of GABA in synaptosomes," *Planta Medica* 60 (1994): 278–79.

22. G. Warneche, "Neurovegatative dystonia in the female climacteric: studies on the clinical efficacy and the tolerance of Kava extract," *Fortschr Med* 109 (1991): 120–22.

23. A. Soulairac and H. Lambinet, "Clinical studies of the effect of the serotonin precursor L-5 Hydroxytryptophan on sleep disorders," *Schweiz Rundsch Med Prax* 77 (1988): 19–23.

24. P. Leatherwood et al., "Aqueous extract of valerian root improves sleep quality in man," *Pharmutcol Biochem Behavior* 17 (1982): 65–71.

25. O. Lindahl and L. Lindwall, "Double blind study of a valerian preparation," *Pharmacol Biochem Behavior* 32 (1989): 1065–6.

26. R. Nave, R. Peled, and P. Lavie, "Melatonin in improving evening napping," Eur J Pharmacol 275 (1995): 213–16.

27. Stolze, "An alternative to treat menopausal complaints," *Obstet Gynecol* 3 (1982): 674.

28. K. A. Hanson and S. Tho, "Androgen and bone health," Semin Reprod Endocrinol 16 (1998): 129–30.

29. R. D. Dickerman, W. J. McConathy, and N. Y. Zacharrah, "Testosterone, sex hormone binding globulin, lipopropteins and vascular disease risk,". *J Cardiovasc Risk* 4 (1997): 363–66.

30. "Anti-Escherichia activity of cranberry and blueberry juices," *N Eng L Med* 324 (1991): 1599.

31. B. Larrson, A. Jonasson, and S. Fianu, "Prophylactic effect of Uva-E on women with recurrent cystitis: a preliminary report," *Curr Ther Resev* 53 (1993): 441–43.

32. H. H. Amin, T. V. Subbaiah, and K. M. Abbasi, "Berberine sulfate antimicrobial activity, bioassay, and mode of action," *Can J Microbiol* 15 (1969): 1067–76.
33. N. Bellamy, W. C. Buchanon, and E. Grace, "A doubleblind randomized controlled study of isoxican versus piroxicam in elderly patients with osteoarthritis of the hip and knee," *Br J Clin Pharmacol* 22 (1986): 1495.

Chapter Ten

1. C. Bailey, *Smart Exercise*, (New York: Houghton Mifflin, 1994), 17.
2. G. Sheehan, *Running and Being* (New York: Simon and Schuster, 1978).
3. Alice Feinstein, ed., *Training the Body to Cure Itself* (Emmaus, Pa.: Rodale Press, 1992), 3.
4. Ibid..
5. Baylor College of Medicine Office of Health Promotion, Vitality, Vim, and Vigor: Six steps to more energy (Baylor Plaza, Houston: Baylor College of Medicine Office of Health Promotion).
6. B. Johnson, *Living Somewhere Between Estrogen and Death* (Dallas: Word Publishing, 1997), 57.
7. Feinstein, *Training the Body to Cure Itself*, 19.
8. Ibid., 221.
9. Ibid.

Chapter Eleven

1. Life Application Bible (Wheaton, Ill.: Tyndale House, 1988), 2070.
2. R. Russell, *What the Bible Says about Healthy Living* (Ventura, Calif.: Regal Books, 1996), 141.

Chapter Twelve

1. A. Marsh et al., "Bone mineral mass in lactovegetarians and omniverous adults," *Am J Clin Nutrition* 37 (1983): 453–56.
2. L. Cohen and R. Kitzes, "Infrared spectroscopy and magnesium content of bone mineral in osteoporotic women," *Isr J Med Sci* 17 (19$1): 1123–25.

3. G. E. Abraham and H. Grewal, "A total dietary program emphasizing magnesium instead of calcium," *J Repro Med* 35 (1990): 503–7.
4. W. S. McKane et al., "Role of calcium intake in modulating age related increases in parathyroid function and bone resorption," *J Clin Endocrinol Metabol* 81 (1996): 1699–703.
5. NIH consensus conference, "Osteoporosis," *JAMA* 252 (1984): 799–802.
6. M. S. Christensen, C. Hagan, and C. Christensen, "Dose response evaluation of cyclic estrogen \ gestigen in postmenopausal women placebo controlled trial of its gynecologic and metabolic actions," *Am J Obstet Gynecol* 144 (1982): 873–79.

Chapter Thirteen

1. H. G. Koenig, *The Healing Power of Faith* (New York: Simon and Schuster, 1999), 100.
2. L. Dossey, *Prayer Is Good Medicine* (New York: HarperSanFrancisco, 1996), 10.
3. R. Byrd, "Positive therapeutic effects of intercessory prayer in a coronary care unit population," *Southern Medical Journal* 81, no. 7 (1989): 826–29.
4. D. J. Benor, "Survey of spiritual healing research," *Complementary Medicine Research* 4, no. 3 (1990): 9–33.
5. Life Application Bible (Wheaton, Ill.: Tyndale House, 1988), 896.
6. L. Dossey, *Healing Words* (New York: HarperSanFrancisco, 1993), 15.
7. J. Vennard, "Intercessory Prayer," Sounds True Audio, Boulder, Colo., 1996.
8. R. Foster, *Prayer* (New York: HarperSanFrancisco, 1992), 216.
9. Ibid., 200.

BIBLIOGRAPHY

Herbs and Nutraceuticals

Colbin, Annemarie. *Food and Healing*. New York: Ballentine Books, 1986.

Dorian, Terry. *Health Begins in Him*. Huntington House, 1995.

Fugh-Berman, Adriane. *Alternative Medicine*. Baltimore, Md.: Williams and Wilkins, 1996.

Gazella, Karolyn A. *Professional's Guide to Natural Healing*. Green Bay, Wi.: *Impakt Communications*, 1997.

Gladster, Rosemary. *Herbal Healing for Women*. New York: Simon and Schuster, 1993.

Jensen, Bernard. *Foods That Heal*. Garden City, N.Y.: Avery Publishing Group, 1993.

Murray, Michael, and Joseph Pizzorno. *Encyclopedia of Natural Medicine*. Rocklin, Calif: Prima Health, 1998.

PDR for Herbal Medicines. Montvale, N.J.: Medical Economics Company, 1998.

Vogel, H. C. A. *The Nature Doctor*. New Canaan, Conn.: Keats Publishing, 1991.

Prayer

Breathnach, Sarah. *Simple Abundance*. New York: Warner Books, 1995.

Dossey, Larry. *Healing Words*. New York: HarperSanFrancisco, 1993.

Dossey, Larry. *Prayer Is Good Medicine*. New York: Harper San Francisco, 1996.

Foster, Richard. *Prayer: Finding the Heart's True Home*. New York: HarperSanFrancisco, 1992.

God's Little Devotional Book II Tulsa, Okla.: Honor Books, 1997.

Koenig, Harold G. *The Healing Power of Faith*. New York: Simon and Schuster, 1999.

Owings, Timothy. *Hearing God in a Noisy World*. Macon, Ga.: Smyth and Helwys Publishing, 1998.

Hormones

Laux, Marcus, and Christine Conrad. *Natural Woman, Natural Menopause*. New York: HarperCollins, 1997.

Lee, John R. *What Your Doctor May Not Tell You about Menopause*. New York: Warner Books, 1996.

Nachtigall, Lila, and Joan Rattner Heilman. *Estrogen: The Facts Can Change Your Life*. New York: HarperPerennial, 1995.

Humor

Adams, Patch. *House Calls*. San Francisco: Robert Reed Publishers, 1998.

Johnson, Barbara. *Living Somewhere Between Estrogen and Death*. Dallas: Word Publishing, 1997.

Klein, Allen. *The Healing Power of Humor*. Los Angeles: Jeremy Tarcher, Inc. 1989.

Samra, Cal, and Rose Samra. *More Holy Humor*. Nashville, Tenn.: Thomas Nelson Publishers, 1997.

Exercise

Bailey, Covert. *The New Fit or Fat*. New York: Houghton Mifflin, 1991.
Bailey, Covert. *Smart Exercise*. New York: Houghton Mifflin, 1994.

Nutrition

McMillen, S. I. *None of These Diseases*. Grand Rapids, Mich.: Baker Books, 1984.
Russell, Rex. *What the Bible Says about Healthy Living*. Ventura, Calif.: Regal, 1996.

Menopause

Budoff, Penny Wise. *No More Hot Flashes*. New York: Warner Books, 1984.
Greenwood, Sadja. *Menopause Naturally*. Volcano, Calif: Volcano Press, 1992.
Ojeda, Linda. *Menopause Without Medicine*. Alameda, Calif: Hunter House, 1992.
Taylor, Dena, and Amber Sumrall. *Women of the 14th Moon*. Freedom, Calif: The Crossing Press, 1991.

General Interest

Backus, William. *The Healing Power of a Christian Mind*. Minneapolis: Bethany House Publishers, 1996.
Bord, Marcus J. *Meeting Jesus for the First Time*. New York: HarperSanFrancisco, 1984.
Borysenko, Joan. Minding the Body, Mending the Mind. New York: Bantam Books, 1987.

Canfield, Jack et al. *Chicken Soup for the Christian Soul.* Deerfield Beach, Fla.: Health Communications Inc., 1997.

Hager, W. David. *As Jesus Cared for Women.* Grand Rapids, Mich.: Fleming Revell, 1998.

Little, Paul. *Know Why You Believe.* Wheaton, Ill.: Victor Books, 1987).

Mcginnis, Alan Loy, *The Balanced Life.* Minneapolis: Augsburg, 1997.

Palms, Roger. *Bible Readings on Hope.* Minneapolis: World Wide Publications, 1995.

Remus, Harold. *Jesus as Healer.* New York: Cambridge Press, 1997.

Siegel, Bernie. *Prescriptions For Living.* New York: Harper Collins, 1998.

Dr. Ron Eaker is a board-certified Obstetrician and Gynecologist in private practice in Augusta, GA. If you are interested in Dr. Eaker speaking to your group or would like audiotapes of live seminars, call (706)-733-4427 or write:

Healing Triad Talks
c/o Dr. Ron Eaker
2258 Wrightsboro Rd., Suite 400
Augusta, Ga. 30904

Web address: www.holyhormones.md
E-mail: reaker@POL.net

*TAPES $7.00 each

- *Holy Hormones! Approaching PMS and Menopause God's Way- an Introduction*
- *Complementary Approaches to PMS and Menopause*
- *The Healing Power of Prayer*
- *Herbal Remedies*
- *The Healer Within*

NEWSLETTER: "FLASHES"

A quarterly review of heath news, reports, and advances in the world of complementary medicine with a focus on women's health issues. An emphasis is placed on anchoring the information with biblical wisdom and guidance.

*$10.00 yearly subscription.